PROPRIOCEPTIVE TRAINING

A Review of Current Research

Caroline Joy Co, PT, DPT, CHT, CSFA

*Dedicated to my father, **Vicente Chua Co***
(May 12, 1951 to Feb 6, 2000)

Proprioceptive Training

ISBN: 144990467X EAN-13: 9781449904678

Printed in the United States of America

Disclaimer

This book is intended for informational and educational purposes only. It is not meant to provide any medical advice. Many of the product names referred to herein are trademarks or registered trademarks of their respective owners. Care has been taken to confirm the accuracy of the information presented and to describe generally accepted practices. However, the authors, editors, and publisher are not responsible for errors or omissions or for any consequences from application of the information in this book and make no warranty, expressed or implied, with respect to the currency, completeness, or accuracy of the contents of the publication. Application of this information in a particular situation remains the professional responsibility of the practitioner.

Rehabsurge, Inc.'s mission is to support healthcare and education professionals to continue their educational and professional development. Rehabsurge is committed to identifying, promoting, and implementing innovative continuing education activities that can increase and impart professional knowledge and skills through books, audiobooks, or digital e-books based on sound scientific and clinically derived research. The first Rehabsurge continuing education book was published in July 2009.

As a sponsor of Continuing Education (CE) seminars and workshops, we enable professionals to enhance their skills, pursue professional interests, and redefine their specialties within their respective disciplines while earning CEUs, CE credits, or Contact Hours. Offerings include CE books, audiobooks, and digital e-books, all of which are focused on the latest treatment and assessment approaches and include discussions of alternative and state-of-the art therapies.

Rehabsurge exists to provide the latest treatment and assessment approaches to the practicing clinician. The basic proposition of our business is simple, solid, and timeless. When we bring the latest knowledge and skill to our clients, we successfully nurture and protect our brand. That is the key to fulfilling our ultimate obligation to provide consistently attractive books, audiobooks, and digital e-books.

For permissions and additional information contact us: Rehabsurge, Inc.

PO Box 287 Baldwin, NY 11510.
Phone: +1 (516) 515-1267
Email: ceu@rehabsurge.com

Disability Policy

Rehabsurge seeks to ensure that all students have access to its activities. To that end, it is committed to providing support services and assistance for equal access for learners with disabilities. Rehabsurge has a firm commitment to meeting the guidelines of the Americans with Disabilities Act and Section 504 of the Rehabilitation Act of 1973. Rehabsurge will provide support services and assistance for students with disabilities, including reasonable accommodations, modifications, and appropriate services to all learners with documented disabilities.

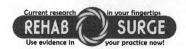

About the Author

Caroline Joy Co, PT, DPT, CHT, CSFA, is a licensed physical therapist and certified hand therapist whose clinical experience includes acute, subacute, home health, and outpatient settings. Her background includes Community-Based Therapy that is designed to help people with disabilities access therapy in their communities using predominantly local resources. She is the President and CEO of PTSponsor.com, an online resource

for U.S. hospitals and clinics that seek to sponsor and hire foreign-trained rehabilitation therapists. She specializes in hand therapy through an integrated approach that includes education, counsel, and exercise. She is also certified in functional assessment for work hardening and work conditioning.

Co is also the President of Rehabsurge, a continuing education company and a contracting agency. Her past affiliations include Long Beach Medical Center, Horizon Health and Subacute Center, and Grandell Therapy and Nursing Center.

Co was a professional speaker for Summit Professional Education, Cross Country Education and Dogwood Institute. She received her transitional doctorate from A.T. Still University and her BS in Physical Therapy from University of the Philippines College of Allied Medical Professions. She is licensed in California, Nevada, and New York.

Full Disclosure

To comply with professional boards/associations standards, all planners, speakers, and reviewers involved in the development of continuing education content are required to disclose their relevant financial relationships. An individual has a relevant financial relationship if he or she has a financial relationship in any amount occurring in the last 12 months, with any commercial interest whose products or services are discussed in their presentation content over which the individual has control. Relevant financial relationships must be disclosed to the audience.

As part of its accreditation with boards/associations, Rehabsurge, Inc. is required to "resolve" any reported conflicts of interest prior to the educational activity. The presentation will be scientifically balanced and free of commercial bias or influence.

To comply with professional boards/associations standards:

I declare that neither I nor my family has any financial relationship in any amount occurring in the last 12 months, with a commercial interest whose products or services are discussed in my presentation. Additionally all planners involved do not have any financial relationship.

Caroline Joy Co, PT, DPT, CHT, CSFA

TABLE OF CONTENTS

Course description vii
Course objectives vii
Chapter 1: Define Proprioception and Identify the Body Systems
      which Affect Proprioception 1
    Introduction 1
    Definition of proprioception 1
    Ontogenesis of proprioception 2
    Acquisition of upright stance 2
    Upright stance to early childhood (6 years of age) 3
    Young adult −7 years to puberty 4
    Adult stage 4
    Body systems that control proprioception 5
    Proprioception and rehabilitation 6
Chapter 2: Compare the Results of Recent Research Studies
      Designed to Test the Effectiveness of Proprioceptive Training 9
    Introduction 9
    Does proprioceptive training work? 10
    Active movement/balance training 12
    Passive movement training 14
    Somatosensory stimulation training 15
    Somatosensory discrimination training 15
    Combined/ multiple system training 16
    Conclusion 16
Chapter 3: Common Orthopedic Diagnoses with Proprioceptive Deficits 19
    Introduction 19
    Osteoarthritis 19
    Rheumatoid arthritis 20
    Osteoporosis 24
    High fall risk 24
    Prehabilitation (prevention of injury) 26
    Post athletic injury 29
    Pre-and post-joint replacement 30
    Amputation 36
    Conclusion 37

Chapter 4: Common Neurologic Diagnoses with Proprioceptive Deficits................**39**

    Introduction...39

    Cerebrovascular disease...39

    Traumatic brain injury 41

    Multiple sclerosis 43

    Parkinson's disease..44

    Alzheimer's disease 46

    Cognitively impaired..49

    Dystonia 51

    Chorea 52

    Conclusion...53

Chapter 5: Evidence-Based Treatment Techniques Designed
           to Alleviate Proprioceptive Deficits. **55**

    Introduction..55

    Evidence-based training techniques....................................55

    Virtual reality and gaming console systems........................55

    Robotic rehabilitation 57

    Reduced weight treadmill systems 62

    Vibration therapy..63

    Adhesive taping systems 64

    Motor imagery (mi) 64

    Video and mirror feedback 65

    Prompting techniques..66

    Constraint-induced movement therapy 67

    Sensory integration 67

    Vestibular rehabilitation 69

    Geste antagoniste (sensory tricks).......................................69

    Proprioceptive neuromuscular facilitation 70

    Progressive agility and trunk stabilization (pats)...............72

    Gait and balance training...72

    Unstable surface drills 75

    Plyometrics and agility training 77

    Mind-body therapies 79

    Aquatic therapy...84

    Conclusion...87

References **89**

Appendix **107**

    Examination 107

    Exam Questions:..108

Answer Sheet **113**

Program Evaluation Form **115**

Course description

Proprioception is integral to nearly all daily life functions. Proprioception affects household and leisure activities, work, and sports, and therefore, it is paramount to have a thorough knowledge of the current research on proprioceptive training. Such an understanding makes it possible for physical therapy professionals to design treatment plans that increase patient lifestyle satisfaction while improving clinical outcomes.

This course will provide an introduction to the fundamental principles of proprioception. The material will identify the bodily systems which foster proprioception, investigate the evolution of sensory-motor systems over the lifespan, identify both orthopedic and neurologic populations, which suffer from proprioceptive deficits, and describe evidence-based treatment options for these patients.

Course objectives

1. Define proprioception and identify the body systems, which affect proprioception.

2. Identify common orthopedic diagnoses, which manifest with proprioceptive deficits.

3. Identify common neurologic diagnoses, which manifest with proprioceptive deficits.

4. Compare the results of recent research designed to test the effectiveness of proprioceptive training.

5. Devise evidence-based treatment techniques designed to alleviate proprioceptive deficits.

CHAPTER 1

DEFINE PROPRIOCEPTION AND IDENTIFY THE BODY SYSTEMS WHICH AFFECT PROPRIOCEPTION

Introduction

Human beings use sensory perception to assess the external environment. Sight, smell, taste, touch, and hearing are the principal signal systems that help us determine whether the external environment carries an overt threat to life or limb. Additionally, the intrinsic systems include equilibrium (balance perception) and proprioception. These sensory systems work in tandem to facilitate movement and to control our reactions to environmental stimuli.

Definition of Proprioception

Proprioception is a term derived from the Latin word proprius meaning "oneself" and the word "perception," a term crafted to illustrate the innate sense of coordination of the various limbs of our body. C. S. Sherrington coined the term proprioception in 1906 in a book titled *The Integrative Action of the Nervous System*. Unfortunately, no one can agree what we mean when we use the term proprioception. In a grander sense, the term proprioception refers to the body's conscious awareness of itself but this is not the complete picture. Certainly, proprioception does include conscious awareness of the body in space including limb position sense, active and passive motion sense, and the sense of weight or heaviness. But this is not the whole of proprioception; proprioception also includes an unconscious component part. The proprioceptive system is responsible for maintaining reflexive control of muscle tone and posture. As you read this, your trunk is unconsciously adjusting as your eyes shift and your head turns to read the words. As you turn the page (or click a mouse) your muscles perform a delicate dance of contraction and relaxation and "restful waiting", always prepared to jump into action, without conscious deliberation or direction. These unconscious acts are also proprioception.

Some researchers choose to distinguish between the conscious and unconscious elements in proprioception by labeling the conscious elements as "kinesthesia" instead and reserving the term proprioception for the unconscious elements (Konczak et al, 2009). It is certainly not a universally held definition.

It helps to think of proprioception as the ability of our body to make changes to our movements "on the fly" based on the additional inputs received from our other visual and tactile sensory organs. To put it simply, proprioception refers to our ability to sense our own body part in space at any given point of time. This sounds simple enough, yet without proprioception, one would not be able to do simple things like walking across a room in a coordinated fashion or lifting a glass of water and drinking without spilling it.

Proprioception can be defined as our brain's ability to perceive and coordinate musculoskeletal functions. It is a combination of forward inputs from the brain to the musculoskeletal system and sensory inputs that can help modulate the forward commands. These functions result in accurate movement of our limbs. Proprioception is an integral part of our voluntary muscle control system. Loss of direction and improper judgment of amplitude of movement can result when proprioceptive sensory inputs are missing. Proprioception is an amalgamation of balance, coordinated movement of limbs, and a perception of how our body parts function in relation to one another.

Ontogenesis of Proprioception

Development of neuromuscular control and the ability to stand and walk independently are important landmarks in the growth of children. In the early stages of infancy, babies are confined to mostly a supine position (unless intentionally placed on their tummies), but this position changes when they learn to flip over and gradually acquire mobility by creeping on their stomach, crawling, and finally walking. Achievement of an upright, bipedal stance and learning to walk are perhaps the most difficult stages in the motor development of an infant. These stages, as well as the activities that infants can participate in, lend insight into the development of proprioception. Maintenance of postural balance and balance during locomotion are hugely complex steps in this process. In short, development of proprioception over the life span can be categorized into four stages (Berger, Trippel, Assainte & Zijlstra, 1995) as follows:

Acquisition of upright stance

Infants acquire adequate neck muscle control, enough to stabilize their head, by the age of three months. Control over trunk muscles and limbs are acquired subsequently. Head and neck control as well as stabilization of gaze are considered to be the beginning of acquisition of postural control and proprioception. It has been postulated that the ability of infants to reach for objects in their environment begins with the stabilization of the head and neck joints and that infants learn to use these parts in an articulated manner. That means that the head and neck joints are stabilized independently and that postural control operates in a cephalocaudal (head to trunk) organization mode. This phase lasts until an upright stance is achieved, which is approximately 12 months of age (average age considered; certainly some infants may walk sooner or later).

Upright stance to early childhood (6 years of age)

Once a bipedal stance is achieved, the next stage in development of proprioception involves postural control by acquisition of control over the head and trunk segments as well as limbs. In this stage, when children begin to walk, stabilization of the pelvis is deemed to be

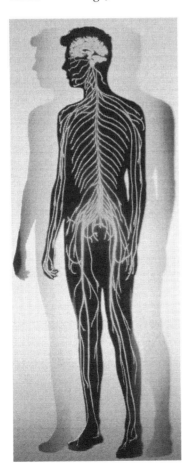

the important step. Walking in one-year old children begins with stabilization of the pelvis and restriction of degrees of freedom for the limbs. In children up to six years of age, the pelvic region stabilizes first during locomotion. Presumably, this allows for restricting the change in the center of gravity and the trunk before the limbs can change their position in order to achieve the desired movement. In this respect, the control of proprioception (postural balance and coordinated movement) originates in a caudocephalic direction. This upward progression is in contrast with the downward progression of proprioception seen in the first phase of development of locomotor and posture control. In this stage, hip movements precede shoulder movements, which in turn precede head movement. This phase is also distinct in that segments of the body are thought to move 'en bloc' in order to 'learn' balance during the early stages of independent walking.

Additionally, sensory cues like visual inputs, vestibular inputs (sensing balance), and other sensory inputs like touch and smell are also important in the development of proprioception in the early childhood. Visual and tactile inputs from surfaces that children come in contact with are particularly significant, and these inputs can be incorporated into the pre-school activities. The development pattern of proprioception is intriguing because of the heuristic (or self-training) mechanisms that underlie it. With an understanding of the mechanism of development of proprioception, it will be possible to design play activities for pre-school children that are centered on the manipulation of various body segments. For instance, since pelvic stabilization is important for locomotion in the pre-school years, it may be useful to incorporate simple dance routines in pre-school activities. Alternatively, games that ask kids to reach out and grab targets that are just beyond their reach may also be helpful. According to the model proposed by Dr. Christine Assaiante (1998), stabilization of the head and neck is task dependent, but pelvic stabilization is an integral part of all activities that children can perform up to the age of 6–7 years. Hence, routines like jumping through tires or dancing with hula-hoops will also help to develop increased proprioceptive control, starting with pelvic stabilization and using the body segments to maintain balance.

Young adult – 7 years to puberty

After the age of six, control of locomotion is thought to proceed in a cephalocaudal manner with increasing degrees of freedom for the limbs. This stage also shows articulated (independently controlled yet coordinated with the rest of the body) operation of body parts. Essentially, the proprioceptive mechanism of the body is now sufficiently trained in order for the individual to gain more and more independent control of distal limbs as well as the pelvic, trunk and head segments of the body. This stage of development of proprioception is also similar to that in older adults.

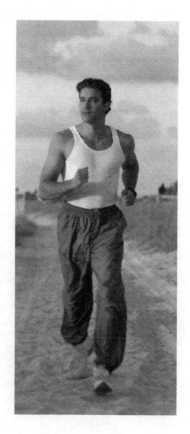

Adult stage

Locomotion in adults is achieved through an articulated operation of limbs and body segments. Essentially, the human proprioceptive control systems are by now well trained to handle complex and/or simultaneous tasks while maintaining postural balance in different situations like walking, reaching out to hold an object, or sitting. The control and coordination of various body parts proceeds in a cephalocaudal manner but with greater degrees of independence for each body part.

Loss of neuromuscular control is also a feature of aging. It would be interesting to understand the correlations between the decline of proprioceptive functions and the development stages (as proposed by Assaiante) in order to understand whether the loss of neuromuscular control is exactly inverse when compared to the developmental stages. If so, there may be a window of opportunity to reverse the aging process by providing exercise-based stimulatory inputs.

Body Systems that Control Proprioception

Proprioception is a function that has been traditionally attributed to the cerebellum. Patients who have undergone brain surgery to remove cerebellar tumors show impaired gait when asked to perform tasks like placing their feet on a target, walking, or walking with weights added to either shank (Giese, Gizewski, Schoch, & Timmann, 2008). However, there is growing evidence that spinal systems may be involved in proprioception as well (Bosco & Poppele, 2001). An in-depth analysis of research on proprioception showed that proprioceptive modulation of movements is controlled by a complex and flexible interplay between biomechanical sensors present in the limbs, motor cortex, and the spine. Features of movements like broad directional tuning, representation of global limb position, kinematics, and common coordinate system for recording spatial information in the cerebellum, sensory cortex and the dorsal spinocerebellar tract (DSCT) are evidence in support of the spino-cerebellar model for control of proprioception.

In fact, dynamic sensory inputs from visual as well as other tactile senses are important for proprioception and accurate movement (Mutha, Boulinguez, & Sainburg, 2001). Volunteers in a trial were asked to reach out towards a specific target. The target could be manipulated to move either before or after the subjects had started the jump. The resulting change in the trajectory of arm movement was analyzed. Additionally, the researchers also applied a pulse force either in the direction of expected movement or opposing the expected movement. These perturbations were created to understand whether the trajectory is determined by forward commands from the brain and reflexes alone or whether sensory inputs helped to achieve the final desired movement. Results from these experiments showed that visual input was important in adjusting the path of the arm taken to reach the target when presented with difficulties like change in target location or limb hindrance. Movement of the arm was a net result of reflexes (forward commands from the brain to the limb), plus visual sensory inputs thereby allowing for a two-level control model for proprioception.

Balance control in humans is reliant upon three cues: visual, vestibular (semicircular canals in the inner ear that sense change in orientation of the head), and cues coming from the entire muscular system. It is easy to understand the role of the visual and vestibular inputs. Without a sense of our surroundings, it would be very difficult to maintain even a static posture. Likewise, perturbations like tilt of the plane of support (the ground, when standing) are sensed in the inner ear. Proprioceptive control is achieved through a dynamic interaction between the spinal column, cerebellum and sensory input organs like skin, inner ear, and eyes. Although not intuitively obvious, visual input is very important in maintaining balance and posture.

Proprioceptive control therefore appears to be a dynamic and flexible system of feed forward control from the cortex, motor control from the cerebellum as well as the spine, and gain adjustment from the feedback of the sensory systems. This is significant especially for people with amputated limbs or for those who have undergone surgery for brain tumors. The dynamic and flexible nature of proprioception can be exploited to "retrain" the brain to "recognize" and readjust the movement potential of their bodies in such patients. This is the basis for the popularity of proprioceptive training exercises being included in the rehabilitation of patients.

Proprioception and Rehabilitation

Proprioception is a vital component of our locomotor abilities. It involves a dynamic system of maintaining balance and coordination of limbs in static postures as well as when walking and performing other physical tasks. Proprioception is the reason why every physical activity we perform can potentially be executed with precision and grace.

As just discussed, proprioception develops in early childhood when infants learn to manipulate their body sections by stabilizing neck movements, flipping over on their tummies, crawl and gradually progress to an upright stance. Understanding this process is vital in order to design rehabilitation activities for toddlers to help them develop adequate control over their limbs as well as develop kinesthetic intelligence. Moreover, such rehabilitation protocols would also help people born with developmental challenges and those who suffer from dysfunction at a later date in life.

The beauty of the proprioceptive system is that it is a "learned" behavior. The immense flexibility and dynamic nature of this system is the reason why people can perform an amazing range of movements at various stages in life, even in their later years, when physical strength is presumed to be at its lowest ebb. This is an important fact to integrate into our lives since people assume that they cannot learn any physical exercise in their sixties and seventies and actually give up their chance of improving their health at that age, thereby indirectly promoting life-threatening or disabling diseases. Proprioception also helps us to adapt to various environments that require a large range of movements with varying degrees of freedom.

Although not immediately apparent, loss of proprioception brought on by disease or trauma can make even simple actions like walking seem like a Herculean task. The real magic lies in the fact that the same control over our limbs and skeletal muscle systems can be brought back with physical training. Emphasis on balance, direction, and control (contrasted with the greater emphasis on building bulk and strength alone) seem to be the hallmarks of proprioceptive training routines. Therefore, one can use multiple methods to achieve appropriate proprioceptive control over our muscles. These can range from simple routines like a one-leg stand to yoga and T'ai Chi as well as other physical training disciplines. It is possible, then, to devise proprioceptive training protocols to suit an individual's needs, taking into account other factors like specific deficits and age.

Recently, proprioceptive training has shown promise as a significant therapeutic intervention in intractable and debilitating conditions like Alzheimer's disease and Parkinson's disease. Given that drug-based treatments for these diseases are inadequate, early interventions with proprioceptive training may help to improve the quality of life afflicted with these diseases and possibly slow the progression of these diseases. The reversal of depression and related neuropathies for Alzheimer's patients and improvement in balance and gait for Parkinson's patients resulting from physical training routines are particularly significant. These are important outcomes indeed; however, more research is needed to arrive at precise proprioceptive training methods for each of these diseases. Also of interest is the fact that exercise is known to increase the levels of endorphins or 'feel good' neurotransmitter (Sutoo & Akiyama, 2003). A large component of an individual's health and well being also depends upon his or her psychological state, and therefore it is important to harness the "mood elevating" effects of exercise to maintain emotional and psychological health as well.

COMPARE THE RESULTS OF RECENT RESEARCH STUDIES DESIGNED TO TEST THE EFFECTIVENESS OF PROPRIOCEPTIVE TRAINING

Introduction

Given the fact that proprioception is such a key part of motor "command and control", it only makes sense to consider if proprioception can be trained. There are dozens if not hundreds of interventions which lay claim to the ability to provide "proprioceptive training" thus altering proprioception and improving motor control.

One of the complicating factors is the fact that much of proprioception is inextricably linked with movement. This is not so for other senses. It is possible to train hearing (for instance, pitch perception) without requiring any gyrations of the body or limbs. It is possible to train the palate to taste subtle nuances of flavor without movement (once the food is placed in the mouth). But proprioception cannot easily be trained passively. With the exception of vibration training, acupuncture and a few other techniques, most proprioceptive training requires movement. Because of this, it becomes quite difficult to tease out if training improved (as one example) a patient's Berg balance test score because of an improvement in proprioceptive sense or because of an increase in strength, ROM, visual acuity or a host of other factors.

In a 2008 study, Vaugoyeau, Viel, Amblard, Azulay, & Assaiante attempted to make that distinction with a test that measured how subjects were able to maintain static posture in a single session. In this study, subjects were blindfolded (thus eliminating sight) and then were asked to stand on a surface that was slowly tilted. The degree of tilt was kept lower than the detection threshold of the vestibular canals, in an attempt to eliminate vestibular sense as a source of information. The challenge presented by the change in surface was gradual and subtle and the predominant response seemed to come from the proprioceptive systems. Stabilization of the head and trunk were noted, and the researchers found that in the absence of visual and vestibular cues, proprioception was instrumental in maintaining static posture.

Does Proprioceptive Training Work?

In 2014, Aman et al published a systematic review looking at many of the recently performed studies, which purported to examine proprioceptive training. In order to ensure that the studies included in the systematic review were actually measuring what they said they were measuring, the studies all had to meet a seemingly low threshold for criteria. Each study had to:

- Measure proprioception, both pre and post study, using a quantifiable method

- Provide an intervention specifically designed to alter or improve proprioception

- Use an outcome measure that was appropriate for testing somatosensation and/or kinesthesia.

It's quite telling that out of over 1,284 articles examined, all of which purported to research the training effects of proprioception, only 51 studies (with 1,854 subjects) met those basic standards. Within those 51 studies, five basic "types" of training were used in an attempt to alter proprioception: (1) active movement and balance training; (2) passive movement training; (3) somatosensory discrimination training; (4) somatosensory stimulation training; and (5) combined training or multi-system training techniques. Each of these five categories of treatment can be further broken down into multiple methods of training used in the field. For instance, the Somatosensory Stimulation category includes studies, which investigated the effects of electrical stimulation, magnetic stimulation, acupuncture, thermal stimulation and movement training, and various types of vibration training.

Obviously, clinicians and researchers must believe there is more than one effective method to train proprioception. (See the sidebar for a breakdown of the techniques.) Just because a training technique is popular in the field (or, for that matter, used as a tool within a study) does not mean that the technique actually does what it is designed to do: enhance proprioception.

Research Training Methods Used to Alter Proprioception

In Aman et al's 2014 systematic review on proprioception, the authors found 17 different types of techniques used by researchers to try and alter proprioception. They broke these into five main categories and then further classified them as follows.

Within the Active Movement/ Balance Training Category, interventions that were used required participants to actively move a limb, a limb segment, or their entire body. Within this category, researchers used the following training methods:

- Balance training (Diracoglu et al., 2005; Hilberg et al., 2003; Risberg et al., 2007; Kerem et al., 2001; Eils and Rosenbaum, 2001; Eils et al., 2010; Kynsburg et al., 2006; Kynsburg et al., 2010; Panics et al., 2008; Sekir and Gür, 2005; Badke et al., 2011; Westlake and Culham, 2007)

- Multi-joint active movement (Röijezon et al., 2009; de Oliveira et al., 2007; Hocherman et al., 1988; Hocherman, 1993; Robin et al., 2004; Wong et al., 2012; Casadio et al., 2009a; Jan et al., 2008; Lin et al., 2007; Lin et al., 2009; Jacobson et al., 1997)

- Single-joint passive versus active movement (Beets et al., 2012)

- Multi-joint passive versus active movement (Wong et al., 2011; Kaelin-Lang et al., 2005)

Within the Passive Movement Training Category, interventions that were used typically required some type of passive motion apparatus and focused either on single-joint (wrist or knee) or multi-joint movement (thumb movement or assisted reaching via robotic arm). Within this category, researchers used the following training methods:

- Single joint passive movement (Carel et al., 2000; Dechaumont-Palacin et al., 2008; Ju et al., 2010)

Within the Somatosensory Stimulation Training Category, interventions that were used_included various forms of stimulation that was geared exclusively to somatosensation. Within this category, researchers used the following training methods:

- Electrical stimulation and rehabilitation therapy (Yozbatiran et al., 2006)
- Magnetic stimulation (Struppler et al., 2003)
- Acupuncture (Liu et al., 2009)

- Thermal stimulation and movement training (Chen et al., 2011)
- Vibration (Rosenkranz et al., 2008; Rosenkranz et al., 2009; Chouza et al., 2011; Haas et al., 2006; van Nes et al., 2004)
- Vibration with active movement training (Cordo et al., 2009; Conrad et al., 2011)
- Vibration with balance training (Merkert et al., 2011)
- Vibration and rehabilitation therapy (van Nes et al., 2006; Ebersbach et al., 2008)

Within the <u>Somatosensory Discrimination Training Category</u>, training focused on the subjects' ability to discriminate between opposing somatosensory stimuli. These discrimination tasks included haptic discrimination (e.g., active exploration of objects with the hand), tactile discrimination (of textures), wrist joint velocity discrimination tasks, and wrist or ankle joint position discrimination. Within this category, researchers used the following training methods:

- Somatosensory discrimination (Carey and Matyas, 2005; Lynch et al., 2007; Mace et al., 2008; Carey et al., 1993; Bakan and Thompson, 1967)

Within the <u>Combined/Multiple Systems Category</u>, interventions which were used included either multiple components of the three main categories mentioned above or utilized multi-sensory approaches. Within this category, researchers used the following training methods:

- Multisensory stimulation and active movement training (Klages et al., 2011)
- Multisensory stimulation and balance training (Missaoui and Thoumie, 2009)
- Somatosensory discrimination and active movement training (McKenzie et al., 2009)

Active movement/balance training

Almost half of the studies included within this noteworthy 2014 systematic review fell into the Active Movement/ Balance Training category. It is interesting to note that those studies employing some version of **active** joint position sense training showed the largest effect sizes of all the studies (a larger effect size makes it possible to find significance within a study). In short, these studies appear to suggest that therapists are best advised to spend their time providing interventions, which encourage active movements, and not creating passive training scenarios. Overall, balance regimens, which lasted 6 weeks or longer were the most popular and showed the greatest potential.

In the studies, which examined reaching, or grasping, **robot-assisted training** sessions (guided by a computer program) showed great promise. In one study, after only 10 hours of training, patients with late effects of stroke were able to reduce upper extremity reaching or grasping error by 80%. This same concept, only with the lower extremities, was promising for patients with osteoarthritis: Goal-directed actions (for instance, tapping on certain targets) were improved through the provision of visual feedback.

Interestingly, these robotic programs are guided by computer programming designed to provide as much assistance as required executing a task. This method, known as online haptic feedback or "assist-as-needed force", appears to be very useful in eliciting proprioceptive training. Researchers also examined the question of how to best notify patients of error during training – in other words, would it better to provide an auditory signal or a visual one to indicate the need to make a correction? Their research showed it was essentially a wash. Both auditory and visual feedback led to improvement, but neither was significantly superior to the other.

Another active therapeutic regimen, which was tested for effectiveness, was the training of "joint position sense". Multiple research teams looked at whether patients could improve their ability to match joint positions through ongoing practice with feedback. The results were significant, with subjects showing the ability to reduce error by 15-63% with multiple training sessions.

One study used active movement training to try to solve an intractable problem. This study was designed to look at chronic neck pain patients. In this study, patients were positioned with an apparatus on their head, which allowed them to control movements of a ball by making minor movements with their head and neck. By the end of the training, subjects were able to reduce the error frequency in neck movements by 19%.

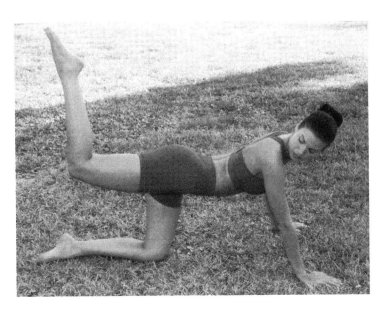

—— *Proprioceptive Training* ——

Active balance retraining remains a popular choice, both in the clinic and in the research field. Many studies included within this systematic review chose to use **"balance training" tasks** as their primary intervention. These balance tasks included sit-to-stand transfers, single and double leg stance activities (with eyes open and eyes closed), standing, walking and jumping on both stable and unstable support surfaces, stair-stepping, and sport-specific drills. All the studies showed that the balance training interventions produced improvement from pre- to post-intervention with a range of improvement spanning from 16% to 97%.

In short, whether the research teams used complicated computer-driven robotics or simple balance training tasks, such as single limb stance, their subjects demonstrated the ability to decrease their movement and positioning errors and increase their proprioception. Active movement training and balance drills worked. It was just a matter of practice and repeated execution.

Passive movement training

Researchers who were interested in the benefits of "passive movement training" used various types of **passive motion apparatus** to determine if the subject could detect passive joint movement and if so, how soon. While all passive motion apparatus were designed differently,

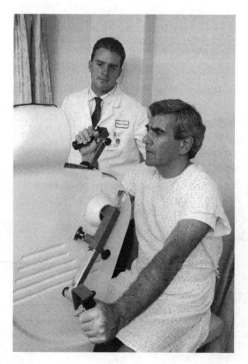

they all worked in a similar manner. The passive motion apparatus was used in order to passively move the subject's arm, say, for instance, the elbow, in order to determine proprioceptive acuity and sensitivity. The researchers were able to determine the exact thresholds where movement became noticeable and then determine if this effect was trainable. Several of the research projects focused on the effects of training a single joint, such as the wrist or knee, while others examined multi-joint movements.

Yes, most studies showed a training effect, although this effect was not nearly as spectacular as the improvement seen with active movement or balance training. All passive motion apparatus studies reported a range of improvements up to 23%, with the exception of Ju et al (2010), which showed a much higher improvement rate (37-47%).

Somatosensory stimulation training

Studies, which looked at somatosensory stimulation, used a wide variety of techniques, including **acupuncture, magnetic fields, electrical stimulation and thermal stimulation**, but the most popular intervention, by far, was **vibration**. Ten studies included within this systematic review applied vibration, some to the muscles, others to the skin and some to the whole body. The studies, which used whole body vibration, were predominantly focused on neurological populations, such as Parkinson's disease or stroke. One such study (Van Nes et al, 2004), showed a significant reduction in center of placement (COP) displacements while standing after receiving only 4 45-second bouts of vibration.

Some researchers chose to combine vibration with active movement or balance training in order to determine the overall or synergistic effect on proprioception. For instance, Merkert et al (2011) combined whole body vibration with functional activities, such as bridging, sitting or standing. The subjects would stand, sit or otherwise position on the vibration plate while performing a functional task (such as standing). This study, which looked at geriatric stroke patients, showed that 3 weeks of training (15 unique sessions) of combined treatment could produce a 61% pre- to post-test improvement in the Tinetti Gait test, which was better than the improvements shown by subjects who only received standard rehabilitation exercises (without vibration).

Interestingly, the duration of vibration used during most studies was quite short, with almost all researchers applying the stimulation between 30-60 seconds at a time. And while the frequencies of vibration used by researchers varied, the most typical frequencies were <10Hz or between 25-30 Hz (for just one example, the Van Nes study used 30 Hz). Researchers who chose to use frequencies under 10Hz did not see the positive results shown with higher vibration frequencies. It is possible that such low vibration frequencies did not induce or excite enough activity in the afferent fibers (found in the muscle spindles) to produce proprioceptive processing. And while most studies held frequencies to under 30 Hz, those that did not (for instance Cordo et al, 2009) showed the most significant functional change. In Cordo's study where vibration frequencies of 60-70Hz were used, stroke patients showed 100% improvement in proprioceptive sense over a period of 6 months. As a rule of thumb, clinicians wishing to see similar changes should make sure to use vibration frequencies greater than 30 Hz.

Somatosensory discrimination training

There are different kinds of sensory discrimination, each worthy of further investigation. The studies, which looked at haptic discrimination, were attempting to determine the ability of subjects to actively explore objects placed in their hand. The studies, which looked at tactile discrimination, were often focused on the ability to differentiate unique textures or shapes or sharpness. Other studies, which focused on **position sense and velocity sense**, tested the subject's ability to differentiate between two joint positions or two speeds of movement. Researchers who focused on the ability to discriminate sensations used a variety of techniques, but they all examined the kind of training effect that could be realized after a series of interventions. While most of the studies examined were small, with correspondingly tiny effect sizes, overall there was a strong trend towards subjects showing improvement in somatosensory discrimination with training.

Combined/ multiple system training

Only three studies looked at what would happen if more than one category of treatment approaches were combined. Of these three, the study by McKenzie (2009) was the most notable. In this study, active movement training techniques were combined with somatosensory discrimination techniques in order to treat patients with focal hand dystonia, such as writer's cramp or musician's cramp. Their unique protocol of treatments resulted in a 90% improvement (for those with writer's cramp) and 22% improvement (for the musicians).

Conclusion

There no longer appears to be any doubt that proprioceptive training can create improvements in proprioceptive dysfunction. This conclusion is supported by the fact that the majority of studies examined in Aman's "study of studies" showed either a moderate or large effect size. This is not unimportant; as any therapist who follows the literature is aware, it is quite difficult to get a team of researchers to state a positive conclusion in most systematic reviews – the effect sizes are just too small for any kind of global statement to be made. Even more remarkable is the fact that well over half (29 out of 51) of all the studies in this review showed an improvement rate greater than 20%.

There is a growing consensus about the type, duration, applicability and scope of proprioceptive training (Aman et al, 2014). First, it now appears that the most effective training programs include somatosensory stimulation as a key component. Incredibly, some forms of somatosensory stimulation (for example whole body vibration) have demonstrated

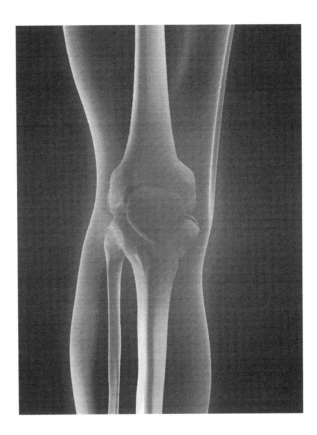

dramatic results within a single session or a few hours of intervention. Therefore, these interventions should never be ignored in the clinic.

Active movements appear to provide a more significant training effect, although a combination of active and passive movements (with and without the provision of exteroceptive feedback) show the largest effect sizes. Longer duration treatments routinely show greater improvements in proprioceptive outcomes, with regimens lasting longer than 6 weeks demonstrated the greatest significance; however, there is little consensus on what the "ideal" training dosage should be. It is important to note that proprioceptive training is not effective for the "neuro" population alone, or for the athlete, or for the post-surgical patient. Proprioceptive training appears to provide value across diagnostic lines.

CHAPTER 3

COMMON ORTHOPEDIC DIAGNOSES WITH PROPRIOCEPTIVE DEFICITS

Introduction

Proprioceptive training has become a standard "go to" treatment for the rehabilitation of patients with many orthopedic complaints. Research has shown benefit with training programs ranging from a single day (Lin et al., 2007) to 6 weeks (Kynsburg et al., 2010). But proprioceptive training is useful for more than just injury or surgery recovery; recent research has demonstrated that there is no "ideal" patient for whom proprioceptive training is required. Rather, many different diagnostic groups can benefit from such programs. Interestingly, the diagnoses that most therapists would classify as most-likely-to-benefit, such as athletic injury and post-joint replacement are not the only populations, which have shown benefit from proprioceptive training. Many other musculoskeletal conditions have also been investigated clinically and shown to benefit from proprioceptive training.

Osteoarthritis

Osteoarthritis (OA) remains the most prevalent joint disorder on the planet; at least 21 million Americans are affected (Olson, Furman, & Guilak, 2012). There are several mechanical factors, which commonly lead to the onset of osteoarthritis; these include age-related joint wear, trauma to the joint structures (cartilage, bone or ligament), and excessive load due to obesity. Of special concern is the fact that obesity is reaching epidemic numbers, a fact, which will only increase the incidence of osteoarthritis, joint replacements and revisions (Lobstein, 2015).

Osteoarthritis brings a host of problems to the table, not the least of which is a series of proprioceptive defects. In a 2012 meta-analysis looking only at the effectiveness of proprioceptive training exercises for the osteoarthritic knee (Smith et al), researchers found that proprioceptive exercises significantly improved the functional status of patients within 8 weeks of training. When the research team compared the effects of proprioceptive-specific training versus a more generalized exercise program, they found that the proprioceptive exercises were more beneficial when looking at tests related to joint position sense, for example, timed walking over uneven ground.

In 2014, a systematic review by Aman et al. supported these findings by demonstrating that the population of musculoskeletal patients, which has shown the greatest benefit and most significant improvement from proprioceptive training, is osteoarthritis, specifically osteoarthritis of the knee. In all the studies included in Aman's systematic review, the knee populations had the greatest improvement overall, with an increase in the parameters ranging from 42%-61%.

Rheumatoid Arthritis

Rheumatoid arthritis (RA) is not nearly as common as osteoarthritis. Only about 0.5-1% of the general population have rheumatoid arthritis diagnosis; this translates to somewhere in the neighborhood of 1.5-2 million Americans (CDC, Nov 6, 2014). Scientists are finally starting to understand the underlying pathophysiology of rheumatoid arthritis. Rheumatoid arthritis can best be understood as an immune-mediated inflammatory disease. Rheumatoid arthritis is a disease wherein chronic and repetitive inflammation of joints is observed, and systemic inflammation is also a feature. In contrast to "wear-and-tear" osteoarthritis, which is typically focused on 1 or 2 joints, rheumatoid arthritis is a polyarthritis, meaning that it affects a minimum of 5 joints in the body. Rheumatoid arthritis is labeled as polyarticular with more than five joints affected or pauciarticular if four or fewer joints are affected by the condition.

Rheumatoid arthritis destroys much of the joint's integrity. Both groups of arthritis patients, osteoarthritis and rheumatoid arthritis, show a significantly elevated fall risk compared to patients without arthritis, and both populations show impaired balance, impaired mobility, a reduced activity level and a lower fall efficacy score (Hill et al, 2013). Around 65% of both osteoarthritis and rheumatoid arthritis patients also report one or more falls over a 1-year period. While patients with rheumatoid arthritis do worse on most tests than their colleagues with osteoarthritis, these differences only show significance during the maximal excursion portions of the Limits of Stability test.

Rheumatoid arthritis (RA) can produce altered gait and biomechanical stability in both children and adults. Although rheumatoid arthritis is treatable with drugs, it can still lead to persistent neuromuscular defects. Delay in neuromuscular development, laxity in joints and ligaments, as well as general and specific growth deficits can result from early-onset rheumatoid arthritis (juvenile rheumatoid arthritis). Such deficits often mean that children are restricted in their physical activities, which, according to the World Health Organization definition, is considered as a disability. Over time, patients may learn to subconsciously hold the affected limbs in a position of comfort, usually in a flexed state, further altering the body's ability to protect and manage its limbs.

In a case reported by Myer and colleagues (2005), a 10-year-old girl with a case history of juvenile rheumatoid arthritis was treated with a specialized neuromuscular training protocol (see sidebar for details). The patient wished to participate in soccer and basketball, however, this raised concerns for her joint health. Extensive kinetic and physical measurements showed that she had diminished neuromuscular ability in her lower limbs. The ability to attenuate force or maintain stability and postural control and strength in the lower extremities of her body was compromised by juvenile rheumatoid arthritis. She therefore risked aggravating joint inflammation if she were to participate in physically demanding sports without prior neuromuscular strengthening interventions. In order to achieve this, physicians adopted a specialized neuromuscular training intervention protocol, which is discussed in depth in the sidebar.

This case report goes on to show that it is possible to progressively train and utilize proprioceptive and graviceptive training to build muscle strength that has been compromised by an inflammatory disease. In all the exercise routines used, the intensity of training was adjusted according to the pain reports provided by the patient. Visual feedback with video recordings and regular communication with the trainers helped the patient to overcome the joint and muscle disabilities caused by juvenile rheumatoid arthritis .

The successful outcome of these training schedules became apparent over time. The patient reported progressive reduction of pain in the knee joints. She reached a stage wherein there was no pain experienced before, during, and after exercise. Neuromuscular training helped the patient achieve near normal gait when compared to age and gender matched normal children. Increased muscle strength was also a significant outcome. The patient's right hamstring strength increased by 85% and the left by 115% (when compared to her pre-training measurements). Similarly her quadriceps femoris muscles also showed strength gain, 18% on the right side and 26% on the left (again as compared to her strength measurements before the neuromuscular training). Improvements in postural balance were also observed after the patient underwent the training protocol prescribed. Single-leg balance when measured on a stabilometer showed 56% and 46% improvements in the right and left leg, respectively.

Juvenile rheumatoid arthritis can result in limiting physical activity in children even after the joint inflammation is controlled by drugs. It is just one of many diseases which can alter proprioception in individuals. The effectiveness of proprioceptive training is clear from this case study. Rehabilitation in the form of exercises and routines designed to strengthen muscles and retune the force exertion behavior can indeed help to overcome these limitations enough to enable the patient to participate in higher intensity physical activities. This report also points out that joint and muscle rehabilitation can be achieved with low-impact specialized neuromuscular training that focuses on improving load distribution and multi-planar movements.

Sample Proprioceptive Training Protocol for JRA

In a case reported by Myer and colleagues (2005), a 10-year-old girl with a history of juvenile rheumatoid arthritis was treated with a specialized neuromuscular training protocol. The protocol consisted of:

Warm-up:

Warm-up consisted of walking with intervals of running on the treadmill. Variations like walking on an incline to increase flexion of hips were also progressively introduced. The aim of this stage was to bring about symmetrical contribution from both legs. Asymmetric contributions were assessed by the sound of footfalls on the treadmill. These exercises were also adopted to equalize range of motion (ROM) for both the patient's legs. Speeds were gradually increased so that the patient experienced the least pain per iteration. If pain was reported, backward treadmill running was used for warm-ups.

Landing stance correction:

The patient needed to have adequate control in the lower extremities when performing landing jumps. Prior tests had shown inequality of limb use and high ground reactions forces. The patient was reliant more on non-muscular structure like ligaments, subchondral bone, and articular cartilage to reduce forces acting upon joints more than the leg muscles. Since abnormal joint loads and poor dissipation of the load have been known to cause osteoarthritis in normal athletes, it was imperative to get the patient to reduce joint load during landing as well as well as teach her correct knee and hip flexion techniques. In order to achieve this, the patient was asked to go through the following series of jump techniques: Jump and hold end position for 30 seconds, box drop and hold, broad jump, broad jump vertical, and overhead jump in a progressive manner. The difficulty levels were increased as the patient achieved more and more control. In the landing techniques, the patient was asked to mentally map her knee joint as a single plane joint (instead of a freely rotating ball and socket joint) in order to reduce coronal load. The idea was to make her visualize her movement to restrict knee flexion to the sagittal plane and eliminate sudden unanticipated jerks or loads on the knee joint when jumping and landing.

Unanticipated Training:

At a stage when the patient had gained sufficient traction over her knee joints, an element of unanticipated training was added to the routine. This was done in order to achieve "muscle-dominant" neuromuscular facilitation. In other words, sudden changes forcing reactionary loads on the patient's leg joints (within safe limits) were expected to enable her to respond almost involuntarily. This was necessary to bring her training protocol akin to maneuvers that she would encounter in her sport-specific training. In order to do that, the patient was put through sprinting and cutting drills, routines she was not preconditioned to perform.

Limb Symmetry:

The patient was found to exert unequal forces with her legs in the jumping and landing exercises. In order to correct this imbalance, she was asked to perform single-leg hops so that each leg could be trained to operate independently of the other. Single-leg hop-and-hold exercises forced the patient to balance independently on each leg.

Core Strengthening:

Core strengthening is essential for correct posture and balance. The juvenile rheumatoid arthritis patient in this case was asked to perform core-strengthening exercises that included double-leg and single-leg squats, single-leg stands, and multiple-angle lunges. Exercises on unstable surfaces like Swiss ball, BOSU Pro Balance Trainer, and Airex Balance Pad were taught to the patient to progressively strengthen not only her legs but also hips, back, and abdominal muscles. Although the patient experienced late-onset muscle soreness, this was countered by introduction of stretching exercises at the end of each session.

Osteoporosis

The National Osteoporosis Foundation (NOF) estimates that a total of 54 million adults over 50 are affected by osteoporosis and low bone mass (Wright et al, 2014). Osteoporosis is a systemic disease characterized by a loss in bone mass and an increased fracture risk. Bone remodeling is a life-long process. In osteoporosis, the skeleton is still capable of laying down bone; in other words, there is no incapacitation of the body's ability to mineralize. However, the aging process creates a perfect storm of factors, which make it less likely for the body to retain its bone mass. After menopause, estrogen levels decline, which — coupled with a reduction in weight-bearing and muscle-stressing activities — reduces the body's bone formation capacities.

The World Health Organization has established a standard measurement for osteoporosis by comparing Bone Mass Density (BMD) with young adult women who are at the age of peak bone mass.

+ Normal bone mass = t score > -1

+ Osteopenia = t score between -1 and -2.5

+ Osteoporosis = t score < -2.5 (or >2.5 SD below the young adult mean)

In the U.S alone, there are 250,000 hip fractures and 500,000 spinal fractures each year and — worse — 50–70% of women do not recover fully after hip fracture. Twenty-five percent will die within the first year post-fracture. For those who make it through the year, the consequences of osteoporotic fracture include diminished quality of life, decreased functional independence, and increased morbidity and mortality.

Proprioceptive training can contribute to a decreased fracture risk by maintaining or improving bone density and improving balance, leading to a decreased risk of falling. However, any exercise program designed to retard the rate of bone loss (or increase the rate of bone growth) must consider what kinds of exercise will produce the best results. The factors most likely to be in consideration include: the frequency and duration of the activity, the ground reaction forces (GRF) created during the activity, the amount of muscle-bone tension created during the activity, and the patient's age at the time of activity.

High Fall Risk

Each year, 1 in 3 community-living adults over the age of 65 years falls (American Geriatrics Society, 2001). Falls are even more prevalent among elderly residents of nursing homes: one study found that approximately 1.5 falls occurs per nursing home bed-year (Vu et al, 2006). Following a hip fracture, frequent and injurious falls are even more common; a 2007 study observed an elevated fall risk in 92% of participants in the year following hip surgery (Lloyd et al, 2009). Among a range of age adjusted risk factors in this study were lower strength, deteriorated balance, and decreased physical activity levels. Results of a 2010 study on postoperative falls in an orthopedic inpatient unit showed that most falls were bathroom related and occurred while the patient was unassisted (Ackerman et al, 2010). Nineteen percent (*n*=13) of patients were injured as a result of falling. Independence is one of the major factors affecting quality of life among the elderly; increased fall risk while unassisted (and subsequent fall efficacy) can have significantly deleterious effects on quality of life.

Falls among the elderly create a huge societal cost due to their frequency, associated morbidities, and high social and economic costs, especially when it causes increased dependency and/or the beginning of living life in an institution. Researchers have reported that elderly women have a higher propensity for falls because of their relative lack of lean body mass and muscle strength, a higher prevalence of chronic-degenerative diseases, and exposure to risky domestic activities. Falls are not just *caused* by poor proprioception, but they can also have a deleterious *effect* on proprioception. While most trauma results in minor clinical consequences, it can occasionally have drastic results, including the onset

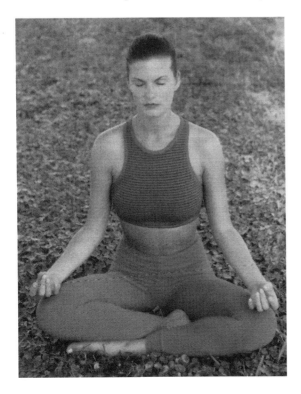

of frailty, thus leading to inpatient treatment and increasingly long stays in health care facilities (Saverino et al, 2006). Fall risk is of particular concern among individuals with orthopedic health issues. Fall efficacy and health problems related to falls represent a persistent problem among the frail elderly (Rubenstein, 2006). A negative loop can develop after a first fall, one comprised of fear, self-directed immobility, weakness, loss of bone density and future falls.

Proprioceptive training can be implemented in the training of patients at high fall risk with resultant improvements in joint stability and muscle control. Geriatric health is a concern, especially since the elderly often live alone or in institutions where care can be sporadic. In the elderly, maintenance of mental health, in addition to physical health, is a primary concern. It is therefore interesting to understand whether physical training, and especially proprioceptive training like yoga and T'ai Chi, can exert positive psychological and physical benefits in patients prone to fall risk (Vu et al, 2006). Vu et al (2006) identified a number of potential intervention strategies including environmental assessment, evaluating and modifying assistive devices, changes in medication, educating the nursing home staff, gait assessment and training, and exercise programs. Gait training and exercise programs are of particular relevance, as the positive effects of these interventions can be generalized to elderly persons living independently as well as those in retirement communities and nursing homes.

Prehabilitation (Prevention of Injury)

Bressel and colleagues (2007) compared the performance of college female basketball players, gymnasts, and soccer players for static balance as well as dynamic balance. Static balance test included double leg, single leg, and tandem stances on stiff as well as compliant surfaces. The players were asked to perform multi-directional single-leg reaches while being supported on a unidirectional tethered support. Interestingly, women basketball

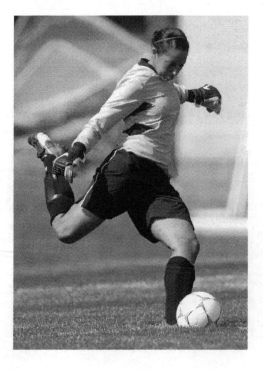

players scored the maximum errors on the static balance tests. The balance errors shown by gymnasts were 55% lower than those shown by basketball players. In dynamic balance tests, soccer players demonstrated 7% higher scores than basketball players. These researchers have attributed these differences to lack of some sensorimotor challenges in basketball players rather than any other benefit conferred unto gymnasts and soccer players by their overall sport activity. In other words, basketball players probably require additional proprioceptive training to compensate for balance errors in static and dynamic postures (Bressel, Yonker, Kras & Heath, 2007). Given that training methods for each sport are inherently different, the apparent differences in proprioceptive abilities can be explained. However, comparative studies shed light upon the fact that enhancement of proprioception is important even for people who are engaged in vigorous physical activities.

In another interesting experiment, McGuine, Greene, Best, and Leverson (2000) tested a similar hypothesis. A set of 210 high school basketball players (119 male and 91 female), 15–17 years of age, was tested for balance and posture maintenance. These players were tested before the game season and had not suffered ankle or knee injuries before participating in the study. All the players were asked to stand on one leg (three trials lasting for 10 seconds each for each leg with eyes closed and open) and their postural sway was monitored. A compiled score (COMP score) of all trials was considered as the sway value. The players were monitored throughout the season to assess ankle injuries severe enough to make the players miss matches. Interestingly, players who sustained injuries had a higher COMP value (2.01 +/- 0.32) as compared to that of players who did not sustain incapacitating ankle sprains (1.74 +/- 0.34) (McGuine et al., 2000). However, regression analyses pointed to a good correlation between a high COMP score and incidence of ankle injuries in these players. The frequency of ankle injuries was seven times greater in players with poor balance as compared to the frequency of injuries in players with good balance.

The natural conclusion from these observations would be to conclude that preventative proprioceptive training should be used to pre-empt ankle injuries. In other words, it is tempting to assume that a reduction in the frequency of ankle sprains and injuries should result from interventions with proprioceptive training. But is this assumption valid? This hypothesis was tested in another study with a larger cohort of teenage basketball players. McGuine and Keene (2006) in University of Wisconsin, Sports Medicine Center provided proprioceptive training to 373 high school players. Incidence of ankle injuries and sprains was seen to be lower in the intervention group (6.13 %) as compared to the standard athletic conditioning exercises group (9.9 %). Furthermore, the risk of repetitive ankle sprain injuries was reduced by 50% in the intervention group when compared with control groups.

So it appears that proprioception can be enhanced by using specific training exercises. In fact, not only is it possible to tweak this neuromuscular sensory system, it is also useful to provide specific modulatory inputs periodically to derive significant health benefits from proprioceptive neuromuscular training. Consider the following case studies. In a study conducted on female soccer players over a two-year period, 1,041 players were asked to include proprioceptive training exercises prior to soccer sessions (Mandelbaum et al., 2005). The control group consisted of 1,905 age and skill matched players who engaged in traditional warm-up sessions before playing soccer. Over a two-year period, the occurrence of anterior cruciate ligament injury was reduced by 88% in the proprioceptive training group. In the second year of follow-up, the incidence of ligament tear injuries was 74% less in the group trained with proprioceptive interventions as compared to the control group. Clearly, proprioceptive training was instrumental in preventing injuries in professional athletes.

In another study conducted with women handball players from Hungary (Panics et al., 2008), proprioception training enhanced the judgment of the knee joint position in these players. Twenty young female handball players were asked to perform proprioceptive exercises. Nineteen players were included in the control group. Periodic assessments before, during, and after the season showed that players who received proprioceptive training scored better on the joint position assessment tests than the control group of players. The increased sensory perception was perhaps instrumental in preventing injuries.

Interestingly, pre-emptive proprioceptive training may be more important for female athletes than male. Joint flexibility studies have showed a gender-based bias in the perception of knee joint motility. Rozzi, Lephart, Gear, and Fu (1999) showed, in their study of male versus female basketball and soccer players, that women have greater knee joint laxity than men. They construed this to mean that the perception of motion when extending the leg is slightly slower in women than in men. Although women show a

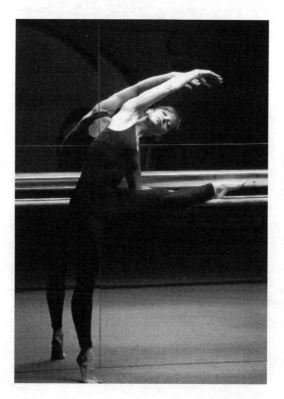

greater ability to balance on one leg, they display a time lag in sensing knee joint movement. This lack of proprioception seems to be compensated by greater activation of the hamstring muscle (as compared to men) when completing tasks like landing after a jump. However, since the knee joint proprioception seems to show a lag, there exists a possibility that women athletes may be insensitive to stresses that impact their knee joints. This phenomenon is likely to leave room for further injury. Hence, there may be a greater need to train female athletes with specialized proprioceptive exercise routines.

As shown by all of these studies, pre-habilitation proprioceptive training programs seem to be effective in preventing injuries. These results reinforce the plasticity of the neural control systems that govern our sense of balance and dynamic force adjustment to maintain balance and posture.

Post Athletic Injury

If proprioceptive training can prevent the primary onset of injuries, is it safe to assume it can also prevent the reoccurrence of injuries? In other words, can training be used to rehabilitate damaged systems and prevent future athletic incidents? Any soft-tissue injury, whether due to repetitive stress, disease or soft tissue damage, will affect the proprioceptive systems of the body. So can these injuries be rehabilitated and the body "made whole" again?

In a 2015 systematic review and meta-analysis, Schiftan et al examined the current state of evidence on the effectiveness of training the proprioceptive systems of athletes with recurrent ankle sprains. Their study showed that proprioceptive training produced a significant reduction in ankle sprain incidence for athletes, irrespective of ankle injury history. In other words, the proprioceptive training was effective for both prevention of ankle sprain and for reoccurrence of ankle sprain, although it was much more beneficial for those with a prior history.

According to Chinnavan et al (2014) a group of subjects with grade-II anterior cruciate ligament tears were divided into two groups to help answer this question. One group of injured subjects participated in a traditional non-operative ACL injury program. The other group was trained using the same exercises plus wobble board drills. After three weeks of 4x/week sessions, the group, which added the wobble, board drills performed much better than the control on the outcomes, including standing balance and timed tests.

Proprioceptive training is routinely recommended for players recovering from injuries. As just one example, in a study involving 20 football players who had previously undergone bilateral ankle sprains, it was seen that ankle sprain injuries resulted in postural sway and ankle repositioning errors (Fu & Hui-Chan, 2005). Passive ankle repositioning errors at five degrees to the plantar flexion were assessed for injured players as well as for age-matched control group of uninjured players. When both groups were subjected to the Sensory Organization Test, the research team found that the injured players displayed greater postural sway and ankle positioning errors. These results suggest that specific proprioceptive training is required during rehabilitation of athletes post-injury.

Pre- and Post-Joint Replacement

As the population ages and arthroplasty surgical techniques become more finessed, the demand for total joint replacements will continue to rise – and with it, the need for successful pre and post-surgical training regimes. By 2030 more than 570,000 primary total hip arthroplasty procedures will be performed annually in the U.S., representing an increase of 174% from 2005 volume. And according to the same source, nearly 3.5 million primary total knee arthroplasty cases will be performed by 2030, a staggering 673% increase (Kurtz et al. 2009). Total ankle surgeries remain much less mainstream, but they continue to grow, with surgeries doubling between 2010 and 2011, according to the American College of Foot and Ankle Surgeons (2012).

Proprioceptive deficiencies are repeatedly reported in the literature for total hip, knee and ankle populations. Sadly, as many as one out of every four patients who undergo a total hip or knee replacement surgery sustains a fall within two years of their surgery (Jogi et al, 2015) and these falls are not benign. The repercussions of a single loss of balance episode can reverberate through the patient's body, household and the healthcare system at large. The cost of falling is astronomical when it leads to a loss of independence, a loss of livelihood, or even a loss of life.

Patients who fall become fearful of falling and that fear (coupled with the results of learned immobility) often produces a self-fulfilling prophecy. Individuals who have suffered a fall routinely demonstrate reduced physical capacity compared to their non-fall counterparts. In fact, those individuals who fear falling score lower on performance measures, grip strength tests, and timed up and go (TUG) tests. They even score lower than their non-fearful peers on objective measures like bone density. Clearly, prevention is the key; if patients who undergo lower extremity joint replacements can be prevented from falling in the first place, the downward cycle of fear and immobility will not initiate and perpetuate.

But can proprioceptive training programs even produce meaningful change for the total joint replacement population? Gstoettner et al (2011) attempted to answer this question, looking first at the patient scheduled for surgery, during the pre-operative period. Their study examined whether proprioceptive training, provided prior to the surgical intervention, would improve balance and functional activities of daily living (ADLs) after surgery. The study participants received six weeks of proprioceptive training prior to their scheduled knee replacements, while a control group did not. All the participants were then retested six weeks s/p arthroplasty surgery and the conclusions were clear. The training group showed significant improvement in stance stability (balance), stiffness, pain and other scores, when compared to the participants who received no proprioceptive training before their surgery. The training worked.

But the benefits of proprioceptive training are not just present when performed in a pre-operative capacity; they are also present when post-operatively as a supplement to a more traditional strength and range of motion rehabilitation protocol. Liao et al (2013) assessed the effectiveness of augmenting a standard total knee replacement program with additional balance drills. A control group was used to determine if the addition of balance specific training to a traditional program would make any meaningful difference. After 8 weeks of training, the group which received supplemental training showed a significant improvement in 10-meter walk times and in the Timed Up and Go Test. The augmented training also improved functional scores on outcome tools like the WOMAC.

Reference for Score: Roos EM, Roos HP, Lohmander LS, Ekdahl C, Beynnon BD. Knee Injury and Osteoarthritis Outcome Score (KOOS)--development of a self-administered outcome measure. J Orthop Sports Phys Ther. 1998 Aug;28(2):88-96.

WOMAC Score

INSTRUCTIONS: This survey asks for your view about your knee. This information will help us keep track of how you feel about your knee and how well you are able to do your usual activities.

Answer every question by ticking the appropriate box. If you are unsure about how to answer a question, please give the best answer you can.

Symptoms - These questions should be answered thinking of your knee symptoms during the last week.

1. Do you have swelling in your knee?

     Never   Rarely   Sometimes   Often   Always

2. Do you feel grinding, hear clicking or any other type of noise when your knee moves?

     Never   Rarely   Sometimes   Often   Always

3. Does your knee catch or hang up when moving?

     Never   Rarely   Sometimes   Often   Always

4. Can you straighten your knee fully?

     Never   Rarely   Sometimes   Often   Always

---

5. Can you bend your knee fully?

    Never   Rarely   Sometimes   Often   Always

Stiffness - The following questions concern the amount of joint stiffness you have experienced during the last week in your knee. Stiffness is a sensation of restriction or slowness in the ease with which you move your knee joint.

6. How severe is your knee joint stiffness after first wakening in the morning?

    None   Mild   Moderate   Severe   Extreme

7. How severe is your knee stiffness after sitting, lying or resting later in the day

    None   Mild   Moderate   Severe   Extreme

Pain

1. How often do you experience knee pain?

    Never   Monthly   Weekly   Daily   Always

What amount of knee pain have you experienced the last week during the following activities?

2. Twisting/pivoting on your knee

    None   Mild   Moderate   Severe   Extreme

3. Straightening knee fully

    None   Mild   Moderate   Severe   Extreme

4. Bending knee fully

    None   Mild   Moderate   Severe   Extreme

5. Walking on flat surface

    None   Mild   Moderate   Severe   Extreme

6. Going up or down stairs

    None   Mild   Moderate   Severe   Extreme

7. At night while in bed

    None   Mild   Moderate   Severe   Extreme

8. Sitting or lying

    None   Mild   Moderate   Severe   Extreme

9. Standing upright

    None   Mild   Moderate   Severe   Extreme

Function, daily living - The following questions concern your physical function. By this we mean your ability to move around and to look after yourself. For each of the following activities please indicate the degree of difficulty you have experienced in the last week due to your knee.

1. Descending stairs

    None   Mild   Moderate   Severe   Extreme

2. 2. Ascending stairs

    None   Mild   Moderate   Severe   Extreme

For each of the following activities please indicate the degree of difficulty you have experienced in the last week due to your knee.

3. Rising from sitting

    None   Mild   Moderate   Severe   Extreme

4. Standing

    None   Mild   Moderate   Severe   Extreme

5. Bending to floor/pick up an object

    None   Mild   Moderate   Severe   Extreme

6. Walking on flat surface

    None   Mild   Moderate   Severe   Extreme

7. Getting in/out of car

    None   Mild   Moderate   Severe   Extreme

8. Going shopping

    None   Mild   Moderate   Severe   Extreme

9. Putting on socks/stockings

| None | Mild | Moderate | Severe | Extreme |

10. Rising from bed

| None | Mild | Moderate | Severe | Extreme |

11. Taking off socks/stockings

| None | Mild | Moderate | Severe | Extreme |

12. Lying in bed (turning over, maintaining knee position)

| None | Mild | Moderate | Severe | Extreme |

13. Getting in/out of bath

| None | Mild | Moderate | Severe | Extreme |

14. Sitting

| None | Mild | Moderate | Severe | Extreme |

15. Getting on/off toilet

| None | Mild | Moderate | Severe | Extreme |

For each of the following activities please indicate the degree of difficulty you have experienced in the last week due to your knee

16. Heavy domestic duties (moving heavy boxes, scrubbing floors, etc)

| Never | Rarely | Sometimes | Often | Always |

17. Light domestic duties (cooking, dusting, etc)

| Never | Rarely | Sometimes | Often | Always |

Thank you very much for completing all the questions in this questionnaire.

Liam and colleagues do not stand alone in their conclusion. Jogi et al (2015) came to a similar conclusion when they compared the effects of balance training to a standard home health treatment session during the 5 weeks s/p total hip or knee replacement. In their investigation, one group of subjects was treated with ROM and strength training exercises while another group received the same treatment with the additional of 3 simple balance exercises. After 5 weeks of training, the patients who received the supplemental training scored significantly better on both the Berg Balance Scale and the Timed Up and Go tests.

The ankle is synovial hinge joint formed by the juncture of three bones: the talus, the tibia and the fibula. Primary arthritis is less common in the ankle joint than other joints of the lower limb, but arthritis brought on second to trauma is frequent (Gougoulias, Khanna, & Maffulli, 2009). Because of these weight-bearing forces, it is injured often, sometimes traumatically. Unlike the hip and knee, the ankle is often brought to the need for surgery because of a trauma, such as a rotational fracture or a recurring, severe ligamentous tear, not primary osteoarthritis.

The ankle is biomechanically complex, much more so than either hip or knee. It is subjected to the highest compression and weight bearing force per inch than any of the joints in the human body (Thomas & Daniels, 2003). This means that any "replacement" to the ankle joint is equally complex to fashion. But unlike the gold standard surgery of the past (the ankle fusion), the surgically replaced ankle can be trained proprioceptively. Research has shown that both land and aquatic training programs can improve proprioception in patients with ankle instabilities early during rehabilitation (Asimenia, Paraskevi, Polina, Anastasia, Kyriakos, & Georgios, 2013). As total ankle patients progress from early rehabilitation to late rehabilitation, the emphasis shifts from strength and range of motion to agility, plyometrics and reaction time. Earlier generations of ankle implants were not viable for any sort of return to sport. The current (third) generation of ankle prostheses is allowing better pain relief, fewer gait abnormalities and better return to function, but "playing sports" is still not in the cards for most post-op patients. However, patients who wish to start walking for fitness or start participating in low impact recreational games, like cycling, swimming and golf, should first participate in a proprioceptive training regimen to ensure their preparedness for such activities.

When one of the joints of the lower extremity (hip, knee or ankle) is replaced, the therapist automatically assumes that balance training may be in order. But proprioceptive training is much more than mere "balance" training of weight-bearing joints. This becomes obvious when the shoulder joint is considered. Like other joints, shoulders need replacing. Shoulder replacements are typically prompted by degeneration of the joint structures – usually through osteoarthritis or rheumatoid arthritis — or through a trauma, such as a fracture of the humeral neck or head.

Total shoulder arthroplasties are on the rise. In 1998, only 19,000 total shoulders were performed, while in 2008, that number more than doubled, to 47,000 shoulder replacements (Kim, Wise, Zhang, & Szabo, 2011). For the first time, the number of total shoulder arthroplasties now exceeds the number of hemiarthroplasties performed in the United States. Part of this jump is due to the approval of the reverse total shoulder procedure by the Food and Drug Administration in 2003.

Proprioceptive training of the shoulder, a non-weight bearing joint, looks quite different than proprioceptive training of the lower quarters, but it is still designed to improve body/spatial awareness of the surgical limb during functional tasks, and to enhance postural awareness. After surgery, patients should be taught to incorporate functional exercises into their exercise regimes, which challenge the body's ability to predict and react to signals from the shoulder. Eventually, this might include use of equipment like the Body blade or activities like wall pushups performed on an unstable surface.

Amputation

Over 65,000 amputations are performed each year in the US alone – and more than 1.7 million Americans are living with the loss of a limb (Statistic Brain Research Institute, 2013). Amputations are – by definition — traumatic. Patients who suffer through the loss of a limb must then suffer through a spatial paradigm shift as well. Their bodies no longer look or feel like the bodies, which existed pre-amputation. They roll differently in bed. They require strange new patterns to rise to stand. In other words, after an amputation, balance and proprioceptive retraining are an inherent requirement.

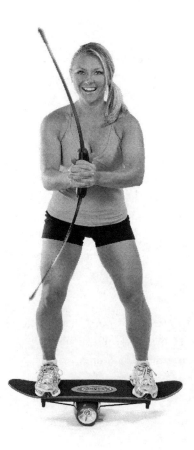

For many years, however, researchers have focused on training proprioceptive tasks with little real-life applications for the amputee. For example, quiet stance has been a common outcome measure for researchers looking to study the effects of proprioceptive training for lower limb amputees. But quiet stance is only one of dozens of proprioceptive deficits present after a lower extremity amputation. Any training regimen following an amputation should include dynamic drills designed to elicit anticipatory postural reactions during walking, reaching, turning the head, and other combination tasks. In addition, dual-processing drills (balance drills which require thinking while doing something else) should be considered a front-line defense against the proprioceptive dysfunction present in amputees.

Conclusion

The orthopedically impaired client is the bread-and-butter of the physical therapy industry and many of these clients are presenting with proprioceptive deficits. However, proprioceptive training is not just for those who are already injured. Importantly, improvements in balance and proprioception made through training regimens have been shown to reduce risk of injury in the future (McGuine et al., 2000; McGuine & Keene, 2006). Therapists working with both orthopedic and neurodiagnostic populations can find ideas for appropriate treatment techniques in Chapter 5.

CHAPTER 4

COMMON NEUROLOGIC DIAGNOSES WITH PROPRIOCEPTIVE DEFICITS

Introduction

Proprioceptive training is not appropriate only for the patient with orthopedic injuries or post-surgical complaints. If anything, this method of training is even more applicable for the neurologically involved populations. However, in order to provide beneficial treatments, it is vital for clinicians to understand the dynamic interplay between the central nervous system and periphery in order to devise therapeutic interventions for patients with neurological events (like TBIs and CVAs) and neurodegenerative diseases (such as Alzheimer's or Parkinson's). Proprioceptive training regimens created for neurologically impaired clients are typically comprised of active multi-joint exercises or whole body movements. Balance drills are limited only by the clinician's imagination, although many of the most popular regimens are discussed in the material to follow. Mind-body techniques, such as yoga and T'ai Chi, have successfully made the transition from holistic programming to proprioceptive training tool. Even the pool, in the form of aquatic exercise or aquatic therapy, has made a strong showing for neurologically impaired clients, allowing balance training a safe environment in which to fail. In the material, which follows, the reader will be shown multiple neurologically compromised conditions, which would benefit from proprioceptive training.

Cerebrovascular disease

In the US alone, over 7 million people have suffered a stroke… and lived. Cerebrovascular disease is the third most common cause of death and the leading cause of serious disability in the United States. Stroke rehabilitation is complex because of the many complications and impairments of function that can follow a cerebrovascular accident, not all of them due to the neurological deficit induced. Weakness or paralysis is the predominant problem in stroke recovery, but the maladaptive compensatory manifestations of spasticity are often a greater challenge in the longer term. Impaired proprioception and balance, together with loss of sensation, results in falls and injury and is often an impediment to therapeutic exercise. The cognitive and emotional alterations that follow cerebrovascular disease can also impede rehabilitation, but may be worsened by the effects of immobility or reduced mobility, as are the many medical complications that attend stroke.

The topic of proprioceptive training for patients who have suffered cortical strokes has been well investigated. Across 16 studies included in a 2014 systematic review, cerebrovascular disease patients saw an average of a 42% improvement in function when treated with appropriate proprioceptive training (Aman et al, 2014). 100% of the studies which used some form of proprioceptive retraining program for the upper extremity showed a significant improvement after treatment.

Proprioceptive training regimens can now include the assistance of mechanical and/or robotic devices (Swinnen et al, 2014; Van Delden et al, 2012), whole body vibration instruments (Pozo-Cruz, 2012), partial body-weight treadmills (Ribeiro et al, 2013), adhesive taping regimens (Grampurohit et al, 2015) and even virtual reality and gaming console systems (Saposnik et al, 2011). Of all the techniques used by researchers, somatosensory training seemed to show the greatest promise, resulting in the most dramatic improvement. Of all the somatosensory techniques used, vibration training stood out from the crowd, with one study showing a 100% improvement in upper extremity function after 6 months of rehabilitation (Cordo et al., 2009).

Much of the effort of stroke rehabilitation is focused upon improvement of balance and prevention of falls. It is important for therapists to realize that the fear of falling often forestalls or limits physical therapy in the post-stroke period even more than any actual injury produced by the fall. Some researchers have begun to ask whether balance training for the cerebrovascular disease population should not take place in a more forgiving environment... namely the therapeutic pool.

There are now dozens of studies, which specifically compare the benefits of balance training on land versus balance training in the water for the patient s/p cerebrovascular disease. As just one example, Park and coworkers (2011) studied 34 patients who were partially ambulatory 6 months or more after stroke. Of these patients, 22 received aquatic therapy and 12 land-based exercises. Six sessions per week, 35 minutes in length, were carried out for 6 weeks. The land-based regimen consisted of the following maneuvers: strengthening lower trunk stability using the upper extremities; walking back and forth, right and left and standing still; tilting the pelvis anteriorly and posteriorly in the sitting position; stretching the arms forward, downward and to the side while seated; standing with both feet together and exchanging a ball with the therapist; and lifting and lowering the heels with feet as wide apart as tolerated.

Exercises in 33-35°C water involved maintaining balance while standing on a board, bending and spreading the hip and knee joints as slowly as possible while standing on the board, walking while wearing a flotation cuff, a bicycling movement with a water-noodle between the legs, standing on the balance board with eyes closed while wearing the flotation cuff, and jumping in the pool with feet together while wearing a cuff.

After 6 weeks of training, both land and water groups showed improved balance and decreased joint position sense errors, but the improvement was significantly greater in the aquatic exercise group and the post-test scores of land and water exercise groups were significantly different. The findings suggest that the joint position disturbance and sensitivity to balance perturbation that contribute to falls in the aftermath of stroke are improved by exercise, and that aquatic exercise is particularly effective in this regard. Obviously, proprioceptive training for the s/p cerebrovascular disease patient works... whether on land or "at sea".

Traumatic Brain Injury

There are about 1.7 million traumatic brain injuries (TBIs) per year in the United States, occurring about every 21 seconds, and over 52,000 people die each year in consequence of their injuries (CDC, 2014). Tellingly, over 33% of all traumatic brain injuries occurred because of a fall; this is more than double the traumatic brain injuries that result due to a motor vehicle accident. Approximately 2 percent of the population has a persistent disability from traumatic brain injuries. These lasting effects include gait disturbance, imbalance, manifestations of spasticity, speech and language impairment, cognitive deficits and adverse alterations of mood, emotions and motivation; all of these impairments may all require treatment and rehabilitation. In short, traumatic brain injury (TBI) is a major cause of death, disability and referral for rehabilitation.

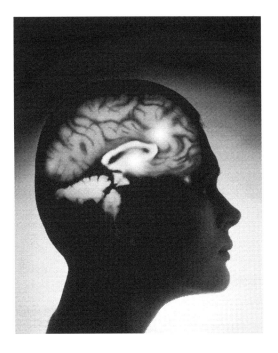

Exercise and rehabilitation has been extensively studied after head injury, with recommendations for treatment based on the Rancho Los Amigos classification system. The Rancho system stratifies head-injured patients by level of response to stimulation as follows:

1. No response;

2. Generalized response not directly to stimulus;

3. Localized response to stimulus;

4. Confused and agitated inappropriate behavior;

5. Confused and inappropriate but not agitated behavior, responds inaccurately to commands;

6. Confused but appropriate behavior and accurate response to commands;

7. Appropriate but automatic behavior, permitting daily activities with minimal confusion;

8. Appropriate purposeful activity and response to environment, functioning memory, and possible depression;

9. Appropriate behavior and purposeful activity with awareness of need for assistance, possible depression;

10. Purposeful, appropriate, modified independence, intermittent depression

Individuals at levels 1-4 are not considered candidates for most types of active proprioceptive training, especially if the training program requires purposeful interaction. Proprioceptive training can be gradually introduced or reintroduced at level 5 or 6 with a structured environment, brief sessions, one-to-one instruction, frequent redirection of attention and simple and repeated commands. Gradual decreases in structure, introduction of activities in which success or failure are possible, increase in complexity of activities, introduction of activities involving cognitive and perceptual skills, involvement in activity planning and goal setting, and socialization are recommended with progression through levels 6-10.

Proprioceptive training programs for the patient with a traumatic brain injury vary tremendously, from vestibular rehabilitation (for mild TBIs such as occur with a concussion) (Gurley et al, 2013) to video-based feedback drills for more low-functioning individuals (Schmidt et al, 2012). Training for this population also makes heavy use of cognitive rehabilitation, both through game consoles, such as the Kinect and through live instruction (Gonzalez et al, 2014).

Multiple Sclerosis

Multiple sclerosis (MS) is the most frequent disabling neurological disease in young and middle-aged European and North American adults (Pugliatti, Rosati, Carton, Riise, Drulovich, Vecsei & Milanov, 2006). According to 2013 statistics from the U.S. Public Health Department, there are approximately 400,000 people suffering with M.S (Statistic Brain Research Institute, 2013). Women predominate over men and onset is most commonly in young adulthood. The disease tends to wax and wane over a period of about 15 years. Patients are often left at that time with permanent neurological deficits, and life expectancy is reduced by 5 to 10 years as compared to the general population.

Multiple sclerosis involves inflammation of — and injury to — the white matter of the brain and spinal cord, but its cause has not yet been determined. Multiple sclerosis, also called disseminated sclerosis, is an inflammatory disease that damages myelin sheath and axons in brain and spinal cord leading to neurological dysfunction. Formation of plaques in central nervous system, inflammation and complete destruction of neurons constitute the pathophysiology of multiple sclerosis. Sites in brain that are most commonly affected are white matter of optic nerve, brainstem, basal ganglia and spinal cord.

The inflammation and multifocal interruption of the myelin sheath that surrounds brain and spinal cord nerve axons prevent the rapid transmission of impulses along the nerve sheath (salutatory conduction), requiring much slower cable-like conduction down the nerve fiber itself. This results in a variety of negative symptoms, such as weakness, sensory loss or incoordination, as well as positive symptoms like pain, paresthesias and involuntary movements. Symptoms may occur in periodic attacks (relapsing form) or continuously (progressive form), with the latter having a worse prognosis.

Neurological symptoms, especially autonomic, visual, motor, and sensory problems, are the most common clinical presentations of multiple sclerosis patients. Patients can have sensory abnormalities like tingling and numbness. There may also be muscle weakness, muscle spasms, and difficulty in moving. Visual problems like nystagmus and optic neuritis, problems in maintaining balance and proprioception are also very common. However, balance and proprioception abnormalities are of major concern in such patients.

Exacerbations are often triggered by intercurrent illnesses such as colds and influenza, and may attend emotional stress and pregnancy. Almost any neurological sign or symptom may be produced by multiple sclerosis, but optic neuritis, spasticity, ataxia and dysarthria, separately or in combination, are the most common. Depression is common and cognitive impairment occurs with progressive disease, while bowel and bladder difficulties are the principal source of disability. Paroxysmal tingling or lancinating pain may occur spontaneously or be triggered by movement (Lhermitte's sign), and symptoms are often worsened by heat (Uhthoff's sign). Women, patients with waxing and waning courses, those with fewer attacks and individuals who develop the disease earlier in adulthood have better prognosis (Cumpston and Compton, 2008).

Although incurable, multiple sclerosis can be treated and symptoms managed by an increasing number and variety of therapeutic approaches, and physical therapy has an important role (Goldenberg, 2012). Studies suggest a high degree of patient and physician interest in alternative and complementary treatments (Schwarz, Knorr, Geiger &, 2008). Physical, occupational and speech therapy have long been used in the rehabilitation of multiple sclerosis patients, and there has been some general evidence of benefit (Thompson, 2000). More recent and specific outcome trials have shown that multidisciplinary rehabilitation improves multiple sclerosis outcome, even in primary progressive cases where drug therapy is not effective (Khan, Amatya & Turner-Stokes, 2011).

Loss of balance control is one of the most feared consequences of multiple sclerosis and it correlates with the severity of the disease (Cameron et al, 2010). Approximately 41% of cases of falls in multiple sclerosis patients have been attributed to balance abnormalities (Peterson et al, 2013). The risk of fall can be largely attributed to the loss of proprioception and inability to maintain postural balance. Even those patients who have normal Romberg and tandem gait tests demonstrate abnormal trunk sway during stance balance tests; in fact, this subtle sign cab be used to aid clinicians in detecting subclinical cases of multiple sclerosis.

A wide variety of training options have been studied and found useful, including resistance or "weight" training (Huisinga et al, 2012), kickboxing (Jackson et al, 2012), aquatic exercises (Barber et al, 2014) and hippotherapy or therapeutic horse riding (Bronson et al, 2010). A systematic review assessing the effects of physical therapy exercises on balance for patients with multiple sclerosis concluded that physical therapy provides significant benefits by enhancing balance and proprioception in those patients who suffered from mild to moderate disability, but not in those with more severe involvement (Paltamaa et al, 2012).

Parkinson's Disease

Another debilitating disorder, which may benefit from proprioceptive training, is Parkinson's disease, a neurodegenerative disease that is on the rise. According to Statista.com (2015), the number of patients with Parkinson's worldwide is on a trajectory to more than double over a 25-year period (from 4.1. million in 2005 to 8.7 million in 20130). Parkinson's disease is characterized by decline in physical, psychological, social, and neurological functions in affected patients. The disease manifests in the form of loss of gait and mobility, tremors in skeletal muscles, postural inability, and loss of balance and coordination. Death of dopamine-stimulated neurons in the motor cortex is responsible for the progressive debilitation seen in Parkinson's disease patients. Since the disease is chronic and progressive, patients gradually lose their ability to perform even simple daily tasks. There are also psychological facets to Parkinson's disease; sufferers are likely to suffer from depression. Although there are drugs available to alleviate specific symptoms of Parkinson's disease, the disease usually progresses to a stage where the patient's movements are severely restricted.

Some researchers argue that these deficits are prompted by changes experienced in the diseased brain's ability to process the barrage of incoming kinesthetic signals. The information, which comes in, is not "read" correctly by the brain and thus the motor action which is generated – which is based on that faulty information — is also faulty.

Patients with Parkinson's disease manifest with atypical patterns of proprioceptive integration. These patients lose spatial awareness of where their limbs are positioned (Zia et al, 2000) and they are unable to accurately estimate limb displacement if their limbs are moved passively (Konczak et al, 2007). Often, patients with Parkinson's complain that their limbs feel heavy (Maschke et al, 2006) and they are unable to adequately regulate grip strength.

Clinically, Parkinson's patients present with many similarities, so much so that therapists have come to identify a "Parkinson's look". Patients with Parkinson's disease have trouble scaling their volitional movements. They depend on visual cues and feedback in order to originate movements and they do not respond "appropriately" to proprioceptive cues, which should signal a change in their motor planning. There is even some evidence that Parkinson's patients have exceptionally poor haptic perception, which is just a fancy way of saying that they can no longer recognize objectives through active tactile exploration of the objects size, texture, shape and so on (Abbruzzese et al, 2014). They move stiffly and intermittently "freeze" during the act of motor planning, especially when presented with non-automated movements (turning a corner, stepping over a doorway threshold, etc.).

Several studies have been undertaken to understand the impact of exercise on Parkinson's disease symptoms in patients. In 2003, two groups of patients with idiopathic Parkinson's disease were taken through a physical exercise program that included strength training as well as balance training. The exercise regimen included high-intensity training like knee flexors and extensors and ankle plantar flexion, as well as balance exercises that selectively included somatosensory cues. These proprioceptive training methods were followed 3 times a week for 10 weeks. The participants were assessed for strength and balance using computerized postural digigraphy as well as sensory orientation tests (Hirsch et al., 2003).

The results showed that both types of training improved the patients' scores on the sensory orientation test. Muscle strength was increased in the group that underwent resistance training, whereas balance was improved in both groups. These results persisted for 4 weeks after completion of the program and bring up interesting possibilities for slowing down the progression of Parkinson's disease, if detected early.

In another study, Parkinson's disease patients with moderately advanced stage of disease (stage 2 and 3 according to the Hoehn and Yahr staging method) were recruited in a gait-training program (Protas et al., 2005). Patients were stabilized with safety harnesses onto treadmills and were asked to walk in all four directions (forwards, backwards, left and right). The training was carried out for an hour, 3 times a week for 8 weeks. At the end of the training period, the participants were assessed for gait, cadence and five-step speed test. Patients in the exercise training group showed significant improvements in gait speed and stride length compared to patients in the control group. The average speed on the 5-step speed test (number of steps completed in a second) also improved for patients who underwent the training program (Protas et al., 2005). Although the effect of the training program on neurological deficits in Parkinson's disease were not assessed in this study, it is still useful to examine, since it highlights the fact that it is possible to introduce physical training to people in early stages of neuromuscular disabilities and regain advantageous control over the voluntary muscles. The study shows that such training protocols may help in reducing the risk of falls and fractures in Parkinson's disease patients. Other studies have also confirmed the fact that gait training is helpful to Parkinson's disease patients in gaining better control over their limbs, especially when administered during the early stages of the disease (Schenkman et al., 2008; Fisher et al., 2008).

According to Aman (2014), whole body vibration therapy is the most studied form of training used for the Parkinson's population. When whole body vibration training is compared to more typical "balance" drills, the results are dramatically better, especially in studies where there is a prolonged period of vibration exposure (Ebersbach et al, 2008). However, more research is certainly called for in this field. There are questions regarding the choice of physical training methods and the exact nature and duration of exercises to be prescribed for Parkinson's disease patients (Goodwin et al., 2008). More investigations and controlled clinical trials are necessary. Nonetheless, the importance of exercise and proprioceptive training in treating early stage Parkinson's disease cannot be ignored.

Alzheimer's Disease

Alzheimer's disease is a debilitating condition wherein patients lose memory, self-recognition, and other cognitive functions, progressively. Worldwide, almost 36 million people have

Alzheimer's or a related cognitive dementia. There are over 5 million Americans living with Alzheimer's; 1 in 9 Americans over 65 has been diagnosed with this disease (Statistic Brain Research Institute; 2015). With this disease, patients gradually lose the ability to perform physical functions on their own. Assisted living facilities are full of patients (over 40% of the census) who may or may not need physical assistance, but who are unsafe to live alone due to the cognitive elements of Alzheimer's disease.

In mice, exercise was found to reduce the deposition of amyloid plaques in the brain. In a mouse model of Alzheimer's disease (TgCRND8 mice), five months of voluntary exercise in mice was sufficient to reduce the amount of amyloid precursor protein by 38% in the frontal cortex, by 53% in the hippocampal area, and by 40% in the hippocampus itself. These results indicate that voluntary exercise can retard the progression of the disease. Interestingly, the cognitive functions of mice also increased simultaneously. When tested in the Morris water maze, the mice that exercised showed reduction in escape latencies. In this study, the reduction in amount of proteolytic fragments of Amyloid Precursor Protein (APP) was seen as early as after only one month of exercise. The proteolytic fragments are indicators of plaque formation. These results suggest that the neuronal mechanisms required to prevent the formation and deposition of amyloid plaques were stimulated by exercise thereby halting the progression of the disease. Although these conclusions are drawn from an animal model and direct extrapolations to human behavior and disease can be derided as a leap of faith, the role of exercise in maintaining neural health is certainly vindicated by the study.

Amnesia or short-term memory loss is an early hallmark of Alzheimer's disease. That being the case, is it rational to expect Alzheimer's patients to observe a daily routine of exercise and sustain it long enough to reap the benefits of exercise? The answer to the conundrum lies in early intervention.

In 1999, Arkin proposed a structured exercise regimen to be executed for elderly people including those suffering from neurological deficits (Arkin, 2003). The exercise program would include aerobic exercises as well as weights and was to be carried out with younger students paired off with an elderly person. Other facets of the training program were language- and memory-stimulating activities. The buddy system would earn the university students credits and facilitate a contact based therapy regime to improve physical and cognitive functions in elderly people. This concept was put into practice with twenty-four Alzheimer's patients (aged 54–88 years) with the help of university students. An exercise schedule that included training for balance, flexibility, aerobic exercises and weight training was designed. Around 16–18 one-on-one sessions and 10 community sessions were conducted per semester for a total duration of 6–8 semesters.

Evaluation of physical fitness at the end of the intervention period showed that the patients had achieved significant gains in their fitness levels as assessed by the six-minute walk test and upper and lower body strength as well as duration of aerobic exercise. Five participants, 86–91 years of age, were able to perform aerobic exercises for 27–45 minutes, which was quite surprising. These five participants were able to undergo the exercise program for the complete duration. Amongst the other participants, nine Alzheimer's patients exceeded the normal range of exercise and five others performed the six-minute walk test just as well as healthy age-matched people.

All the participants in the exercise intervention group showed elevated mood and slower decline in cognitive abilities. These findings are significant in light of the fact that a simple behavioral intervention could be delivered to patients with a highly debilitating disease. Not only was it cost-effective to deliver the therapy, it was also effective in slowing down the loss of mental faculties in patients.

In addition to physical exercise, language-enriched exercise and enhanced social contact in the form of group recreational activities also helps to stabilize the cognitive functions of Alzheimer's patients. These interventions may be useful to slow down the loss of mental faculties when interventions are introduced at early stages of the disease (Arkin, 2007).

Caregivers for Alzheimer's patients can also be involved in providing home-based exercise therapies to Alzheimer's disease patients. In a set of two studies conducted by Teri and colleagues, (1998, 2003), Alzheimer's patients and their caregivers were included in an exercise program designed to provide simple balance and flexibility training to patients with Alzheimer's disease. These studies showed that patients who received the exercise training displayed fewer days of restricted activity as compared to those who received the routine medical care. Patient-caregiver pairs who participated in the exercise intervention group also showed reduced symptoms of depression and a tendency to depend less on institutionalization.

These results are encouraging since the approach is more inclusive. Most long-term illnesses also exact a price from the patient's caregivers as well. Moreover, depression that accompanies neuropathies is also addressed when group therapy sessions or patient-buddy dyads are used for participation in interventions. Improved social contact may help to reduce disruptive social behavior in patients suffering from Alzheimer's disease.

Individuals with neurological dysfunctional syndromes are also prone to lose balance often and suffer from falls, which in turn, can lead to more health complications. Balance training can be introduced as a behavioral modification in such individuals to mitigate the risk of fractures and other impact injuries. Many clinical trials similar to that performed by Hill et al (2009) are underway in an attempt to evaluate the benefits of balance training in people suffering from mild to moderate forms of Alzheimer's disease.

Exercise, though beneficial, is not always effective in treating the cognitive elements of Alzheimer's disease. Patients with cardiovascular co-morbidities do not seem to show the same improvements in cognitive functions despite interventions with exercise. Alzheimer's disease patients with increased cardiovascular risk factors may not show the same benefit from exercise (Eggermont, Swaab, Luiten, & Scherder, 2006).

Cognitively Impaired

It is clear that cognitive functions influence proprioceptive exercise routines and positively affect them. But can physical activity have a reverse influence and increase brain function? This issue was the focal point of a study conducted with 521 individuals residing in retirement communities in the Chicago Metropolitan Area. In a study published in the *American Journal of Geriatric Psychiatry*, Dr. Buchman and colleagues (2008) examined the correlations between daily physical activity and cognitive functions of elderly people not suffering from dementia. In this study, the total daily activity of the participants was measured objectively, using actigraphy instead of relying on self-reports. Cognitive functions were assessed and were found to be directly correlated to the amount of physical activity, also measured objectively. These results indicate that physical inactivity has a negative effect on cognitive functions whereas physical activities can bring about positive cognitive changes in people (Buchman et al., 2008).

But what about patients with cognitive impairment; will they also show cognitive benefits from proprioceptive training? This hypothesis was put to test in a study with residents from nursing homes that showed early signs of dementia (Hornbrook, Stevens, Wingfield, Hollis, Greenlick & Ory, 1994). The researchers hypothesized that; in people suffering from mild cognitive deficits, exercise can help reverse the initial losses in cognitive capability. In the study, the residents were divided into three groups:

- No intervention—This was the control group which did not receive social contact or exercise as an intervention

- Social contact group—This group received a social visit equivalent in duration to those who received the exercise program

- Exercise group—This group of people was asked to perform a set of exercises for thirty minutes per session, three sessions a week for twelve weeks' total duration.

The participants of the study were then asked to perform a clock-drawing test and were assessed for cognitive function according to the Revised Elderly Persons Disability Scale (REPDS). The clock-drawing test showed that the decline in cognitive functions in dementia was slowed down by exercise. The disabilities caused by dementia were reduced with exercise when measured with the Revised Elderly Persons Disability Scale. In some cases, the individuals were able to perform their daily tasks with greater ease when they were taken through an exercise program than before. This indicates that exercise is able to reverse the disabilities induced by cognitive loss in some cases. Importantly, this study also showed that low-impact exercises could be taught to people regardless of age and mental capability. These results are important especially since people tend to ignore exercise as they get older or develop inhibitions and self-doubt about their capability of performing various exercise routines.

In another study with individuals who showed mild cognitive impairment (MCI), a combined approach of group activity planning, assertiveness training, stress management memory training, and motor planning exercise was used to understand whether these therapies could reduce the cognitive deficits (Kurz, Pohl, Ramsenthaler, & Sorg, 2003). Following four weeks of therapy, patients with MCI showed significant improvements in performing daily living tasks and verbal episodic memory. Patients with more advanced cognitive impairments did not seem to respond to the intervention significantly. However, this study highlights the fact that early diagnosis of diminishing mental capability in the elderly may be essential in order to provide therapies like social interactions and exercise. Early intervention may also help to lessen the burden of cognitive impairments, on the individual as well as on society.

One issue that should be thoroughly understood is the effect of a combination of aerobic and anaerobic exercise on brain structures. Sherlock, Hornsby and Rye (2013) cited studies that supported the association of regular aerobic training, i.e., a form of exercise such as "running, walking, swimming or calisthenics strenuously performed so as to cause marked temporary increase in respiration and heart rate" (Merriam-Webster's Collegiate Dictionary, p. 20) with improvements in many aspects of cognitive function, e.g., memory, decision making, problem solving and attention. Furthermore, although few studies have focused on the relationship of anaerobic exercise such as strength training to executive function, the combined prescription of aerobic and anaerobic exercise has been shown to allow participants to improve to a much greater degree than simply engaging in aerobic training. Indeed, the American College of Sports Medicine has endorsed this combination as being "the optimal approach to improve cardiorespiratory fitness, reduce metabolic abnormalities, increase muscular strength and improve functional capacity" (Meredith-jones, Waters, Legge, & Jones, 2011, p. 94). Further, there has been a great deal of research centering on the environment in which this exercise takes place, one that is 'enriched' which, in and of itself, provides a means of mental and physical stimuli that "positively influences neurological processes to become more efficient" (Sherlock et al., 2013, p. 268).

When considering the potential effect of "brain gym" type exercises, it is important to consider the brain's plasticity. When specific neural pathways used by the brain are blocked or damaged, the brain is capable of utilizing alternate means of circumventing those blockages, which results in the establishment of new pathways (Doidge, 2007, as cited by Grosse, 2013), as well as increasing the brain's myelin sheath, thus enhancing transmission speed of electrical impulses and improving its function. In their study of brain health, Cotman, Berchtold, and Christie (2007) found that "exercise sets into motion an interactive cascade of growth factor that has the net effect of stimulating plasticity, enhancing cognitive function ... [and] stimulating neurogenesis" (p. 469). Further, research has found that even those who have already developed symptoms of cognitive impairment can benefit from exercise to improve cognitive function and allow them to be better able to perform activities of daily living (ADL). As Forbes, Thiessen, Blake, Forbes, and Forbes (2013) observed, healthcare providers can confidently prescribe a program of exercise that will not only improve the quality of the lives of their patients, but will also serve to relieve the burden of their caretakers and delay those patients' admission in long-term care facilities.

Dystonia

Dystonia is a neurological disorder in which the patient manifests involuntary muscle contractions resulting in repetitive, slow movement patterns or atypical postures. Some patients with dystonia also demonstrate tremors or other neurological symptoms; almost all cases of dystonia can involve some element of pain. Dystonia can involve only a discrete group of muscles (focal); a group of adjacent muscles (segmental) or it can be widespread throughout the body (generalized). The most common focal dystonia is a disorder known as torticollis. In torticollis, the neck muscles contract and pull the head to one side or (less commonly) pull the head forward or backwards.

Over time, most cases of dystonia worsen or become more noticeable or widespread. The root cause of dystonia is unknown, although there is some consensus that the basal ganglia may be worthy of attention as the source. In patients with dystonia, the brain's ability to appropriately process neurotransmitters seems to be altered and this breakdown in communication creates reverberations in motor planning and feedback. Complicating matters is the fact that diagnostic tests, such as can be performed with magnetic resonance imaging (MRI) devices, show no brain abnormalities. Whatever the root cause, genetics is certainly at play for some forms of the disorder.

Interestingly, most patients who suffer from dystonia can temporarily alter their symptoms by performing certain physical tasks, which provide either proprioceptive or tactile feedback (Abbruzzese et al, 2014). This phenomenon is known as the "geste antagoniste" or "sensory trick." Patients with a focal dystonia, such as torticollis, find that if they perform certain sensory tricks, such as touching their chin, they are able to reduce their dystonic postures or movements, albeit temporarily. It is possible that such sensory tricks cause the individual's brain to recruit additional networks or produce a form of motor-sensory adaptation, but the truth is, no one is sure why it works (Konczack and Abbruzzese, 2013). While therapists and physicians do not know the underlying mechanism of this phenomenon, such proprioceptive training "tricks" can still be taught as a means of sensory modification.

Dystonia can be ever-present or it can come and go, brought on only by certain activities or movements. A common example of a task-specific focal dystonia would be a case of "writer's cramp" or "musician's cramp". Recent research has shown that focal dystonia can be treated with proprioceptive retraining (Rosenkranz et al., 2008, 2009). In a 2009 study, individuals suffering from either musician's and writer's cramp participated in 8 weeks of proprioceptive training which included progressive motor retraining and showed a 10-fold improvement in mean target reaching error (McKenzie et al., 2009).

Chorea

Chorea is a type of dyskinesia, which creates involuntary, abnormal movements. Chorea appears to be caused by excessive activity of the neurotransmitter dopamine in the part of the brain responsible for movement. Chorea manifests as brief, irregular, non-repetitive, and non-rhythmic movements. These movements can appear to flow from one muscle group to another. Often, chorea is paired with athetosis, a movement disorder that manifests with twisting or writhing movement patterns. The most well-known disease in which chorea manifests is Huntington's disease, a hereditary, neurodegenerative disease; however, there are many other diseases in which chorea appears, for instance Sydenham's chorea which can follow rheumatic fever. Chorea can also be associated with certain medications, endocrine or metabolic diseases and some vascular events.

There is no one treatment for chorea. If the chorea was caused due to rheumatic fever, it can be treated with antibiotics to address the infection. If it was caused by metabolic or endocrine imbalances, it can be treated by addressing the root imbalance. If it was caused by medications, the medications can be adjusted or replaced. Unfortunately, the treatment options for the chorea that is associated with Huntington's are basically "supportive" and not therapeutic; Huntington's is not curable.

Unlike Parkinson's patients, who suffer from hypokinesia, patients with dystonia and chorea suffer from *hyper*kinesia. However, both populations suffer from defective or incorrectly processing of proprioceptive signals. The fact that some patients have presented with choreic-like symptoms (also referred to as "pseudo-choreosthetosis") following certain nerve lesions opens up an interesting line of consideration for rehabilitation of the patient (Abbruzzese et al, 2014). Patients with both hypo and hyperkinesia muscular disorders have difficulty coordinating proprioceptive input with visual information, leading to difficulty with activities of daily living. Abbruzzese and colleagues postulated that any rehabilitation of patients with such disorders might benefit from proprioceptive training in order to strengthen the signals necessary for enhanced motor performance.

Conclusion

Almost by definition, the vast majority of neurologically impaired clients are going to present with some element of proprioceptive deficits. Research has shown that proprioceptive training, especially training, which includes sensory modulation and active movement, is beneficial for a wide assortment of populations. And while physical therapists tend to automatically think of proprioceptive training as a synonym for balance training, that is but a small element of the "whole" of proprioceptive training.

EVIDENCE-BASED TREATMENT TECHNIQUES DESIGNED TO ALLEVIATE PROPRIOCEPTIVE DEFICITS

Introduction

Proprioceptive training, as we've discussed earlier, may address agility, balance, strength, accuracy, visual-spatial planning, spatial orientation, coordination or memory skills, amplitude of movement and more. Neurological studies have shown that the proprioceptive system requires a dynamic coordination between sensory inputs and motor control. The most common proprioceptive training programs are discussed, with concrete examples provided for many of the exercise-based techniques.

Evidence-Based Training Techniques

A large number of exercises and other treatments are possible for proprioceptive training; however, a list of commonly used techniques is provided here.

Virtual reality and gaming console systems

Physical medicine and rehabilitation has certainly come a long way from the early days of manual muscle tests. Technology is exploding and training options, which were science fiction even ten years ago, are finding their way into the mainstream. Therapists looking to motivate or encourage participation from clients may need to look no further than virtual reality or game consoles like the Nintendo Wii as the up-and-coming frontier.

Virtual reality

Virtual reality means different things to different people but a helpful way to define it was presented by Weiss et al (2004): Virtual reality is "the use of interactive simulations created with computer hardware and software to present users with opportunities to engage in environments that appear to be and feel similar to real world objects and events."

While many of the virtual reality (virtual reality) systems, which are designed with rehabilitation in mind, are still too expensive to use outside the research lab, the technology continues to trickle down into clinical applications. For instance, computer-based video games, making use of a virtual reality construct, are already in common use.

Virtual reality systems can be clumped into categories to better understand how users are able to make use of the systems (Sveistrup, 2004). The main categories include: immersive virtual reality (which requires a head-mounted display setup) and non-immersive virtual reality (which does not). Immersive systems are very expensive and typically only used in research settings. Non-immersive systems do not require the hardware or software financial outlay and thus are in more common clinical usage. With these systems, users interact with the virtual reality when their movements are captured with a camera-system, another sensor interface, or computer joystick.

Even after the patients completed a traditional rehabilitation program, two-thirds of patients with cerebrovascular disease have deficits in their upper extremities, which significantly impacts function. In a 2011 systematic review, Saposnik and Levin examined the state of the evidence supporting the use of virtual reality as an adjunct to upper extremity rehabilitation programs s/p cerebrovascular disease. Overall, twelve studies were analyzed; eleven of those 12 studies showed additional benefit from the augmented training sessions, with some studies showing a 20% improvement over conventional rehabilitation alone.

Ma et al (2012) compared the training effect of the exact same task (reaching for stationary versus non-stationary balls) when it was performed in the virtual realm versus the real world. The subjects who participated were all diagnosed with Parkinson's disease, a neurodegenerative disorder that impairs reaction time and volitional motor planning. In this study, the researchers found that patients did not react the same when reaching for moving items "in the real world" versus in virtual reality. The subjects who were trained with real moving targets performed differently; they showed better movement speed and synchronization of their trunk and periphery than did the virtual reality group, a finding which may reduce the value of virtual reality as a training tool.

Gaming console systems

Video games have long been a mandatory accessory among teenagers, but it appears that gaming systems have successfully made the leap to skilled therapy modality. Two popular systems which include motion-sensation (the Nintendo Wii and the Xbox 360 Kinect) are both being routinely integrated into nursing home care, "homework" after skilled therapy and even in the clinic.

After a neurological injury or insult, the brain attempts to restructure pathways and to find a new way to do old things. In order for this to succeed, there are multiple factors, which have to fall into place. There has to be a method to obtain immediate feedback. There needs to be a motivational or rewards element. There certainly needs to be a means to repeat tasks as they are learned and mastered and eventually to increase the task difficulty in order to progress. Motion-sensing gaming systems can provide all of these elements by engaging the user in "stories" or plots, assigning scores or points and rewarding some behaviors and not others.

Video games seem especially promising for children and teenagers who need a motivational home program. In a 2005 paper, You et al was the first to describe the actual brain alterations, which occurred in an 8-year old child with cerebral palsy after participating in proprioceptive gaming. The child participated in a specialized video game play for 60-minute sessions, 5x/week for 3 months. The researchers used a functional MRI system in order to provide the first concrete evidence to support their contention that video games do promote neuroplasticity.

Herz et al (2013) examined the effect of video game play on adults with Parkinson's disease. In this study, the subjects used the Nintendo Wii 3x/week for 4 weeks and were then re-tested. The subjects all improved gaming (in quality of life, activities of daily living and motor function) after 4 weeks of and held this improvement for a month after discontinuing the training. In other words, the Wii-based rehabilitation program made it possible for the patients to do more and feel better in as short as 1 month.

Robotic rehabilitation

Robotic rehabilitation is an up-and-coming field, made even more relevant by the dramatic increase in use of robots within the labor industry. Robotics can be used at many points during rehabilitation, from initial assessment of injury to return-to-combat readiness. Robotics is also being used clinically to facilitate gait, to tax balance, and to improve prosthetic interphases.

Swinnen et al (2014) performed a systematic review on the benefits of using robot-assisted gait training for patients who had cerebrovascular disease. There was a great variety in the type of "robotic assistance" used. In some studies, a robotic gait trainer was used; in others a wearable robotic knee orthotic was used. Several other proprietary robotic systems (AutoAmbulator; Lokomat) were also tested. The studies used typical clinically relevant ways to assess whether balance improved; these included the Tinetti test, the Berg Balance Scale, the Timed Up and Go and some postural sway measures. Robotic rehabilitation resulted in definite improvement in balance, as tested by these measures; the question remains, however, whether this level of improvement would have occurred using another (perhaps cheaper) means of balance training. Multiple manufacturers are now designing and crafting intelligent bionic exoskeletons that act essentially as wearable robots in order to benefit patients with significant limitations, such as wounded warriors and paraplegics.

Tinetti Performance Oriented Mobility Assessment (POMA)*

Description:

The Tinetti assessment tool is an easily administered task-oriented test that measures an older adult's gait and balance abilities.

Equipment needed: Hard armless chair
                             Stopwatch or wristwatch
                             15 ft walkway

Completion:

  Time: 10-15 minutes
  Scoring: A three-point ordinal scale, ranging from 0-2.

"0" indicates the highest level of impairment and "2" the individuals independence.

                             Total Balance Score = 16
                             Total Gait Score = 12
                             Total Test Score = 28

Interpretation: 25-28 = low fall risk
                             19-24 = medium fall risk
                             < 19 = high fall risk

Tinetti ME. Performance-oriented assessment of mobility problems in elderly patients. *JAGS* 1986; 34: 119-126. (Scoring description: PT Bulletin Feb. 10, 1993

—— Proprioceptive Training ——

Tinetti Performance Oriented Mobility Assessment (POMA)
- Balance Tests -

Initial instructions: Subject is seated in hard, armless chair. The following maneuvers are tested.

1. Sitting Balance
Leans or slides in chair   =0
Steady, safe   =1   _____

2. Arises
Unable without help   =0
Able, uses arms to help   =1
Able without using arms   =2   _____

3. Attempts to Arise
Unable without help   =0
Able, requires > 1 attempt   =1
Able to rise, 1 attempt   =2   _____

4. Immediate Standing Balance (first 5 seconds)
Unsteady (swaggers, moves feet, trunk sway)   =0
Steady but uses walker or other support   =1
Steady without walker or other support   =2   _____

5. Standing Balance
Unsteady   =0
Steady but wide stance(medial heals > 4 inches apart)
and uses cane or other support   =1
Narrow stance without support   =2   _____

6. Nudged (subject at maximum position with feet as close together as possible, examiner pushes lightly on subject's sternum with palm of hand 3 times)
Begins to fall   =0
Staggers, grabs, catches self   =1
Steady   =2   _____

7. Eyes Closed (at maximum position of item 6)
Unsteady   =0
Steady   =1   _____

8. **Turing 360 Degrees**

Discontinuous steps   =0

Continuous steps   =1   _____

Unsteady (grabs, staggers)   =0

Steady   =1   _____

9. **Sitting Down**

Unsafe (misjudged distance, falls into chair)   =0

Uses arms or not a smooth motion   =1

Safe, smooth motion   =2   _____

BALANCE SCORE: _____/16

- Gait Tests -

Initial Instructions: Subject stands with examiner, walks down hallway or across room, first at "usual" pace, then back at "rapid, but safe" pace (using usual walking aids)

10. **Initiation of Gait** (immediately after told to "go"

Any hesitancy or multiple attempts to start   =0

No hesitancy   =1   _____

11. **Step Length and Height**

Right swing foot does not pass left stance foot with step   =0

Passes left stance foot   =1   _____

Right foot does not clear floor completely with step   =0

Right foot completely clears floor   =1   _____

Left swing foot does not pass right stance foot with step   =0

Passes right stance foot   =1   _____

Left foot does not clear floor completely with step   =0

Left foot completely clears floor   =1   _____

12. **Step Symmetry**

Right and left step length not equal (estimate)   =0

Right and left step length appear equal   =1   _____

13. **Step Continuity**

Stopping or discontinuity between steps   =0

Steps appear continuous   =1   _____

14. **Path** (estimated in relation to floor tiles, 12-inch diameter; observe excursion of 1 foot over about 10 ft. of the course)

Marked deviation   =0

Mild/moderate deviation or uses walking aid   =1

Straight without walking aid   =2   _____

15. **Trunk**

Marked sway or uses walking aid   =0

No sway but flexion of knees or back or spreads arms out
while walking   =1

No sway, no flexion, no use of arms, and no use of walking aid   =2   _____

16. **Walking Stance**

Heels apart   =0

Heels almost touching while walking   =1   _____

                                        GAIT SCORE = _____/12

BALANCE SCORE = _____/16

                TOTAL SCORE (Gait + Balance) = _____/28

{< 19 high fall risk, 19-24 medium fall risk, 25-28 low fall risk}

Tinetti ME. Performance-oriented assessment of mobility problems in elderly patients. *JAGS* 1986; 34: 119-126. (Scoring description: PT Bulletin Feb. 10, 1993

But rehabilitation opportunities with robotic systems are not limited to the lower quadrant. Within the stroke rehabilitation field, training with robotics is taking off, especially training for the impaired upper extremity. Picelli et al (2014) examined the effects of robotic rehabilitation training on impairment of the upper quadrant for patients with Parkinson's disease. They provided 10 sessions, each lasting 45-minutes, 5 days/week, for 2 weeks using a robotic system, which provided repetitive, computer-controlled, mirror-like, bilateral practice sessions. The robot first provided passive movements, then active resisted movements. By the end of the two weeks of training, patients showed a statistically significant improvement in the Fugl-Meyer assessment and in a nine-hole peg test. The authors concluded that the robotic-assisted training showed promise.

—— Proprioceptive Training ——

In 2012, Van Delden et al provided an excellent summary of the clinical applicability of such upper extremity robotic devices, including a ranking system. They looked at 14 robotic systems and evaluated them for such elements as variety of movement patterns, types of training protocols, benefits shown via outcome study and commercial availability. Their results, while not conclusive, do show the growing interest in and market for such upper limb training systems.

Reduced weight treadmill systems

One of the greatest benefits to aquatic rehabilitation is the reduced weight bearing which comes with immersion in water. Buoyancy reduces the amount of compression and impact realized during vertical work in water. But what if you could create this same reduction in weight without having to get wet (or have a pool at your clinic)? The latest craze in gait training is the use of reduced weight treadmill systems also referred to as "partial weight" or even "body weight suspended" treadmill systems. These systems use some form of a harness system to support a portion of the patient's body-weight and position the patient over the top of a treadmill in order to facilitate gait. The equipment is just a means to an end – the reduction of body weight – in order to promote gait or locomotive training.

Ribeiro et al (2013) investigated whether such a treadmill system could be used to promote better gait parameters several years after a stroke; they compared the results of training with the results gained from the use of a more common proprioceptive training technique, the Proprioceptive Neuromuscular Facilitation method of gait. Both groups showed some significant improvement after 12 sessions, but neither group stood out as the "definite winner". The patients improved their motor Functional Independence Measure (FIM) and other functional scores and produced a more symmetric gait cycle, however, the speed of gait, stride length and support time did not improve in either group.

Swinnen et al (2012) asked whether patients with multiple sclerosis who were treated using a partial weight treadmill would manifest superior results to those using a traditional treadmill or a robot-assisted system. In this systematic review, the authors found that all three forms of gait training produced improvements in double limb support time, increases in step length and improvement in disability scales, but that none of the systems had distinguished themselves as superior.

Ganesan et al (2014) found that a reduction of 20% of body weight did allow patients with Parkinson's to realize greater benefits from treadmill training than was possible without this technology.

Vibration therapy

Over the last 10 years or so, there has been an upsurge in interest in the use of vibration (both focal and whole body) on neurologically compromised diagnoses such as spinal cord injury, multiple sclerosis, Parkinson's and stroke. Vibration is even getting a second look for its effect on dystonia. There is a renewed hope that if therapists can better understand the effects of such vibratory stimulation on the central nervous system, new training protocols can evolve. Therapists continue to ask whether whole body vibration is superior to focal vibration, whether a short (<1 minute) bout of vibration is superior to a long one, whether a low frequency (<10Hz) was superior to a higher frequency (25-30 Hz) and whether the stimulation should be applied to the skin, the muscle or the whole body.

In 2014, Murillo et al wrote a comprehensive overview of the state of the evidence on use of focal vibration across the field of neuro-rehabilitation. They reported that overall focal vibration was tolerated well, easy to administer and, above all else, effective. Vibration therapy appears to be useful in the treatment of such neurological deficits as spasticity and dystonia.

Vibration studies seem to be well designed overall. Ten studies were rigorous enough to be included within Aman et al's comprehensive systematic review, already discussed above. The studies, which used whole body vibration, were predominantly focused on neuro populations, such as Parkinson's disease or stroke. One such study (Van Nes et al, 2004), showed a significant reduction in center of placement (COP) displacements while standing after receiving only 4 45-second bouts of vibration.

Some researchers choose to combine vibration with active movement or balance training in order to determine the overall or synergistic effect on proprioception. For instance, Merkert et al (2011) combined whole body vibration with functional activities, such as bridging, sitting or standing. The subjects would stand, sit or otherwise position on the vibration plate while performing a functional task (such as standing). This study, which looked at geriatric stroke patients, showed that 3 weeks of training (15 unique sessions) of combined treatment could produce a 61% pre- to post-test improvement in the Tinetti Gait test, which was better than the improvements shown by subjects who only received standard rehabilitation exercises (without vibration).

Interestingly, the duration of vibration used during most studies was quite short, with almost all researchers applying the stimulation between 30-60 seconds at a time. Researchers who chose to use frequencies under 10Hz did not see the positive results shown with higher vibration frequencies. As a rule of thumb, clinicians wishing to see similar changes should make sure to use vibration frequencies greater than 30 Hz.

Ebersbach et al (2008) asked whether vibration training could be superior to a more traditional method of training balance (use of a tilt board) for patients with Parkinson's disease. The results were fascinating. After 3 weeks of twice-a-day sessions, the patients who were trained using whole body vibration showed a 33% improvement in their ability to control the tilt board while those who trained more traditionally actually worsened, showing a 23% reduction in control.

Adhesive taping systems

Adhesive taping has been explored as a method to alter proprioception for patients with neurological deficits and sports injuries for over a decade. Uses of complicated taping systems, like Kinesiotape, have been embraced by Olympic and other elite athletes.

Grampurohit and colleagues performed the first systematic review asking this very question in 2015. They asked whether the use of adhesive taping as a supplemental treatment for patients s/p stroke was a waste of time and money. In their study of 15 research trials, they found only 4 good quality studies. Other than some evidence to support the use of rigid taping systems to reduce pain, there was not enough research to support the contention that adhesive taping affected almost any outcome parameter examined (including range of motion, strength, function, muscle tone, and proprioception).

Motor imagery (MI)

For years, trainers and physical therapists have been telling their sport medicine clients that "mental rehearsal" is as important and useful way to prepare for sporting events as actual physical practice. Motor imagery is nothing more than the mental rehearsal of a movement without actually making any physical movements. It is essentially practicing a task in your mind but stopping shy of executing it with your muscles. In fact, motor imagery of movements has been shown to create the same neural activation in the brain as the actual movements themselves (Gatti et al, 2013)

First the question of appropriateness needs to be resolved. If there is damage to the brain, which negatively affects motor function, would that damage extend to the patient's ability to mentally, rehearse movements, even without physical movements? The answer appears to be that it is still feasible to use motor imagery (motor imagery) with these populations. According to Di Rienzo et al (2014), "motor imagery capacities may not be deteriorated per se by neurologic diseases resulting in chronic motor incapacities, but adjusted to the current state of the motor system".

Patients with cerebrovascular disease, spinal cord injuries and Parkinson's disease feature heavily in the literature. Parkinson's patients are notoriously slow in both mental imagery of a task and in the execution of the task itself. Because of this, many researchers have felt that motor imagery would not be an appropriate way to attempt to train proprioception in this population.

In 2012, Heremans et al published a study on the use of motor imagery in patients with Parkinson's disease. In this study, the team used external cueing as a supplemental tool to aid the patients in performing motor imaging. Their idea was simple. Since the basal ganglia seems to be implicated as a source of bradykinesia in Parkinson's patients, external cueing should be able to be utilized in order to bypass the basal ganglia and activate alternative compensatory networks. This hypothesized benefit of external cueing had already been tested and found sound with patients who showed bradykinesia during gait. Heremans and colleagues wanted to test whether the benefits of external cueing could be extended to proprioceptive training. They tested two types of cueing (auditory and visual) and compared results against no cueing at all. Their findings showed that the application of **visual** cueing by the therapist performed during motor imagery had a profoundly significant effect on the Parkinson's patients to do mental imagery. With the visual cues, motor imaging becomes a more viable option for training proprioception in the patient with Parkinson's. Although there was some benefit seen with auditory cueing, it was nowhere near as profound as was demonstrated with visual cueing.

Video and mirror feedback

The presence of some form of feedback is a hallmark of most proprioceptive training regimens. Feedback is routinely utilized to help improve patients' self-awareness and motor planning and provide input necessary for correction. Feedback can take on many forms (audio, visual and tactile being the most common), but the use of mirror feedback and video-based feedback has received some recent attention.

In a randomized controlled clinical trial, Schmidt and colleagues (2012) asked if 3 different kinds of feedback provided during a daily task would provide identical benefit for the patient with a traumatic brain injury. In this study, they asked their subjects to perform a meal preparation task and compared the results using three kinds of feedback – 1. Feedback provided via a video; 2. Feedback provided via verbal feedback; and 3. Experiential or internal feedback. The individuals who received video-based feedback did much better than those who only received verbal or experiential feedback. It was useful to the subjects to be able to view themselves performing the acts incorrectly while receiving verbal feedback from the researcher.

Assuming that patients find it helpful to view themselves simultaneously while being asked to make corrections, then mirror therapy would seem to be another useful proprioceptive training tool. Hlavackova et al (2009) asked whether the use of mirror feedback would be useful to elderly amputees attempting to improve upright stance using their prostheses. Their results were a mixed bag, but overall mirror therapy was useful in aiding these patients.

Prompting techniques

Patients who receive proprioceptive training can benefit from different kinds of feedback, as already discussed, including verbal feedback. But all verbal feedback is not equal. There are different methods of providing prompts to patients. Two of these prompting methods have been studied to determine whether the use of such specific prompts would alter motor planning. One of the techniques often used in proprioceptive training is referred to as a "constant time delay procedure". The constant time delay is an errorless teaching procedure in which the stimulus control is transferred from a given stimulus situation (e.g., the teacher) to other stimulus conditions. A study by Yilmaz et al. (2007) sought to determine the effect of a constant time delay procedure on the acquisition of rotational skills in children with autism. Using data collected over a 10-week period from four participants, the study showed that using a constant time delay approach was effective in teaching the Halliwick's method of rotational control. All subjects increased their correct rotation skills significantly during the instruction period, with these gains persisting through the other phases of the method.

A second study by Yilmaz and Birkan (2010) on the use of the constant time delay procedure to teach aquatic play skills to children with autism disorder showed a similar benefit. In this study, the authors collected data over a 10-week period from four participants using the single opportunity method as an intervention. The aquatic play skills assessed the patient's task analysis for completing the aquatic kangaroo, cycling, and snake play skills of the patient, showing significant improvements for all participants. Follow-up data collected up to four weeks after the instruction indicated that the subjects maintained the skills taught during aquatic play. Procedural reliability was shown to be high, and the usefulness of the one-to-one teacher-patient ratio was shown to be useful.

Another prompting technique used in proprioceptive training is known as the "most to least prompt". Yilmaz and Birkan evaluated the impact of the most to least prompting on teaching simple progression of swimming skills for children with autism spectrum disorder. Most to least prompting is an errorless teaching technique that requires giving the strongest prompt to students who respond to the teacher correctly. As the student performs the activities independently from the teacher, the strength of the prompt reduces, until the student becomes independent from the cues and is able to perform the activity on his or her own. The participants of this study were three nine-year-old boys with autism, and the results were assessed using a multiple baseline design across all subjects. While none of the participants was able to perform any correct responses during the baseline assessment sessions, the introduction of physical and verbal prompts significantly improved the performance of the participants. Strong procedural reliability for most to least prompting was demonstrated by teachers participating in the study. Most importantly, these improvements were achieved through the limited time made available for the intervention, indicating its possible usefulness in larger-scale studies.

Constraint-induced movement therapy

Constraint-induced movement therapy (CI) is a training tool, which has been in use, typically with stroke patients, for the last generation. In constraint induced movement therapy, the therapist forces the use of the "affected" side by restraining the unaffected side. During constraint induced movement therapy sessions, the patient's unaffected limb is rendered useless by placing it in a sling. The patient is then asked to use the affected limb repetitively to perform very difficult rehabilitation-specific tasks. Constraint induced treatment is often performed intensively over a relatively short period (for instance, daily for 2 weeks).

Stevenson et al performed a systematic review and meta-analysis answering this question in 2012. Their study of studies examined whether constraint induced movement therapy produced equal, worse or better results than other comparable "dose matched" interventions. They were able to identify 22 studies, which met their criteria, and their results were intriguing and conclusive. Constraint induced movement therapy was shown to be superior to other interventions across the board, in all outcomes assessed including: upper limb ability, upper limb motor capacity, Functional Independence Measure (FIM) scores, Motor Activity Log scores and other factors. Constraint induced movement therapy provided more benefit than other treatment options for the stroke victim with some residual movement in their upper extremity.

Sensory integration

Sensory integration refers to the integration and interpretation of sensory stimuli from the environment from the brain. This is also referred to in other sources as sensory processing. Stimuli from the environment are processed as sensations that are received, modulated, integrated into useful information that the brain uses to interact with the environment. This theory was first described by occupational therapist and neuroscientist A. Jean Ayres

(1972), who hypothesized that impairments in sensory integration manifest as difficulties observed in purposeful behaviors. Patients with sensory processing disorder (SPD, formerly known as "sensory integration dysfunction") are unable to organize sensory signals into appropriate responses, leading to dysfunction in performing activities of daily living, lack of motor coordination, behavioral problems, anxiety, depression, and other impacts.

Although the impact of sensory processing disorder on life participation of individuals is recognized, sensory interventions have been inconsistently defined, and thus, interventions have widely varied. Furthermore, most studies on interventions for sensory processing disorder have been limited in size and robustness. Since Ayres described sensory integration dysfunction in 1972, sensory-based therapies have been increasingly used by occupational therapists and other health professionals to treat a wide range of symptoms in children across a wide range of settings, including the home, community organizations, and school.

A systematic review of literature (Case-Smith, Weaver, & Fristad, 2014) found that studies on sensory integration therapy (SIT) for children with autism spectrum disorder (ASD) and sensory processing disorder demonstrated positive effects on the child's individualized goals. Sensory integration therapy was defined as a clinic-based, child-centered intervention that provides play activities and sensory-enhanced interaction to illicit the child's adaptive responses. Sensory integration therapy goals with children suffering from autism spectrum disorder could complement the goals of other interventions and educational programs. Findings suggested that sensory integration therapy could have limited effectiveness if applied in a school context. However, the same review also indicated the need for randomized clinical trials with blinded evaluations and larger samples.

In contrast, sensory-based intervention (SBI), defined as adult-directed sensory strategies to improve behavioral regulation associated with modulation disorders, was found to have almost no evidence of positive effects. The Case-Smith, Weaver and Fristad review (2014) found that studies on sensory-based intervention lacked rigor, and followed widely different protocols. For example, for SBIs using a weighted vest, only one study demonstrated positive effects. Most studies suggested that the weighted vest did not reduce stereotypic behaviors, improve joint attentions, or reduce distractibility. Studies on sensory-based intervention were found to lack blinded evaluation, to have limited description of the intervention and control measures, as well as to have a non-standardized measure, thereby suggesting that the evidence for sensory-based intervention was insufficient to recommend its therapeutic use.

Given the relative lack of comprehensive literature on the effectiveness of sensory-based therapies, their use should be made within the context of specific treatment goals with objectively measurable, attainable and reasonable expectations.

—— Proprioceptive Training ——

Vestibular rehabilitation

Vestibular rehabilitation is a type of therapeutic programming designed around specific exercises with the intent of promoting central nervous system compensation for deficits in the inner ear (the vestibular system). Vestibular rehabilitation has been used for multiple disorders including: benign paroxysmal positional vertigo; Ménière's disease, vestibular neuritis and labyrinthitis. Even patients with concussions have been treated for their resultant vestibular abnormalities with vestibular rehabilitation. In 2013, Gurley et al looked at whether vestibular rehabilitation would be effective in treating the vestibular complaints found in patients with mild traumatic brain injuries (essentially a concussion) and found that it was an effective tool in addressing dizziness, vertigo and imbalance complaints which followed the traumatic event.

Porciuncula et al (2012) asked whether vestibular rehabilitation therapy has been shown to be effective for patients with bilateral vestibular hypofunction. In this systematic review of 14 studies, they concluded that there was moderate strength evidence supporting the use of vestibular rehabilitation to alleviate the complaints associated with vestibular hypofunction. These findings were also borne out by Arnold et al in a systematic review performed in 2015, when researchers asked a similar question for patients with unilateral peripheral disorders.

Geste antagoniste (Sensory Tricks)

Most patients who suffer from movement dystonia can temporarily alter their symptoms by performing certain physical tasks, which provide either proprioceptive or tactile feedback. This phenomenon is known as the "geste antagoniste" or "sensory trick." Patients find that if they perform certain acts (such as touching their chin), their dystonic postures or movements will reduce or cease all together, albeit temporarily (Abbruzzese et al, 2014).

There is limited information on the pathophysiology behind sensory tricks. In fact, not all "tricks" are sensory (geste antagoniste can include variants like imaginary tricks, motor tricks, forcible tricks and reverse sensory tricks) (Ramos et al, 2014). It is possible that sensory tricks cause the brain to recruit additional networks or produce a form of motor-sensory adaptation (Konczack and Abbruzzese, 2013). It is also possible that sensory tricks are able to modulate the abnormal facilitation-to-inhibition ratios in the brain of the dystonic patient (Ramos et al, 2014). No one is sure. Fortunately, just because therapists and physicians do not know the underlying mechanism of this phenomenon doesn't mean that such "tricks" can't be taught as a means of coping with unwanted dystonia posturing. Almost 90% of patients with cervical dystonia (torticollis) reported using such sensory tricks to alleviate their unwanted posturing. Of those, 40% reported marked improvement and 43% reported partial improvement, and only .03% reported no beneficial effect from performing sensory tricks (Patel et al, 2013).

Sensory tricks are usually specific to the type of dystonia being experienced. Therapists looking for suggestions on types of sensory tricks to suggest are directed to the Dystonia Society's website (http://www.dystonia.org.uk/index.php/living-with-dystonia/coping-with-dystonia/sensory-tricks) which provides a comprehensive list of dozens of such sensory tricks, including: Staring at a fixed point, gum chewing, whistling, humming, talking, resting the head against a wall, reading aloud, sucking on a straw or singing. All of the Society's suggestions have been classified by different underlying types of dystonia, including:

- Neck dystonia (Cervical dystonia or spasmodic torticollis)

- Eye dystonia (Blepharospasm)

- Voice dystonia (Laryngeal dystonia or spasmodic dysphonia)

- Mouth or jaw (Oromandibular) dystonia

- Writer's Cramp

- Generalized / abdomen dystonia

- Paroxysmal dystonia

The suggestions are quite specific and – although the Dystonia Society makes it clear that these are anecdotal suggestions – the lists of sensory tricks are comprehensive.

Proprioceptive neuromuscular facilitation

Proprioceptive neuromuscular facilitation (PNF) is one of the most commonly utilized proprioceptive training techniques used today. These functional spiral movement patterns were derived from the work of Sherrington and his successors, individuals who investigated neuromuscular facilitation and inhibition. The myotatic stretch reflex was known to cause muscle contraction when lengthened too quickly, and an inverse stretch reflex to cause muscle relaxation when the tendon is pulled with too much force; the inverse reflex is due to increased inhibition arising from the Golgi tendon organs (autogenic inhibition), and by reducing motor drive to the muscle facilitates its elongation. Opposing sets of muscles at joints were also shown to work in synchrony, those on one side of a joint relaxing to accommodate the contraction of those on the other; this is accomplished by inhibiting the opposing group when a muscle's stretch reflex is activated by stretching the muscle spindle. The muscle spindle's input to the spinal cord activates an alpha motor neuron to complete the reflex, but also inhibits the opposing alpha motor neuron, thereby preventing the co-contraction of both muscle groups (reciprocal inhibition). This co-contraction is responsible for many athletic injuries and is also characteristic of spasticity.

Herman Kabat took these concepts a step further by suggesting that combinations of movements would be more effective in augmenting excitation in weakened muscles and enhancing inhibition in spastic ones, thereby facilitating muscle elongation. Diagonal and rotational movements and movement across several joints and in different planes were developed, chiefly two sets of diagonal flexion and extension movements for the upper and lower extremities, along with a series of contraction and relaxation exercises that facilitate muscle elongation by increasing inhibition, diminish rigidity by rhythmic movement, increase joint proprioceptive input and through slow alternation of agonist and antagonist contraction take advantage of the phenomenon of selective induction, the enhancement of an extensor reflex after a flexor one has been activated and vice versa. These exercises were developed for use on land, but were also eventually also transferred to warm water in order to take advantage of its buoyancy and resistance (Adler, Beckers and Buck, 2007).

PNF patterns are divided into upper and lower extremity patterns. There are also PNF gait and balance patterns. These patterns are classically designated as D1 (Diagonal 1) and D2 (Diagonal 2) patterns. Each pattern has a flexion component and an extension component and all the joints of the limb are involved in each pattern, creating a "functional" movement of the limb, instead of an isolated joint movement.

The D1 flexion pattern starts with the patient positioned in shoulder flexion, adduction and external rotation, supination of the forearm, and flexion of the wrist and fingers. The ending position for D1 flexion is shoulder extension, external rotation, abduction, forearm pronation, and extension of the wrist and fingers.

The PNF patterns of the lower extremities replicate the same patterns as the upper extremity. The D1 flexion pattern for the LE's includes hip flexion, adduction and external rotation, dorsiflexion of the ankle and inversion and extension of the toes. The D2 flexion pattern includes hip flexion, abduction and internal rotation, dorsiflexion of the ankle, and eversion and extension of the toes. The D1 and D2 extension patterns reverse the movements back to the starting position.

In 2014, a group of physical therapists (Sahay et al, 2014) performed a study in which traditional rehabilitation techniques (weight-shifting, weight-bearing, balance and gait exercises) were compared to PNF techniques in patients with transtibial amputations. The PNF group showed better outcomes than the traditional group, with better scores on the Locomotor Capabilities Index and improved gait parameters (stride length, step length and so on).

Progressive agility and trunk stabilization (PATS)

Sherry and Best (2004) conducted a study on hamstring strains and compared a traditional stretching and strengthening program (STST) to a progressive agility and trunk stabilization program (PATS). The traditional stretching and strengthening program program included the following exercises: stationary bike, supine hamstring stretch, standing hamstring stretch, contract-relax hamstrings stretch in standing, sub-maximal hamstring isometrics, and ice. A progression included stationary bike with moderate resistance, moderate velocity walk, supine and standing hamstring stretch, prone leg curls with weights, hip extension in standing with Theraband resistance, non-weight bearing foot catches, symptom free practice without high-speed maneuvers, and ice as needed.

The PATS program involved: Sidestepping, grapevine, steps forward and backward with lateral motion; single-leg stability with eyes open and closed; prone abdominal body bridge with elbows and feet as only points of contact; supine extension bridge and side bridge; ice; progression to increased intensity side step, grapevine, forward/backward, single-leg stability windmill touches (repetitive alternate hand touches), push-up stabilization with trunk rotation starting at top of push-up, lift hand and rotate body upward toward ceiling and alternate; jog in place; PNF trunk pull-downs with Theraband to right and left; and symptom-free practice without high-speed maneuvers.

The PATS program was more effective than the traditional stretching and strengthening program in return to sports and prevention of recurrence. In the first 16 days of return to sport, 54% of the traditional stretching and strengthening program athletes had a recurrent hamstring strain while none of the PATS athletes had a recurrence. Within the first year of return to sport, 70% of the STST group had a recurrence while only 7.7% of the PATS group had a recurrence of a hamstring strain.

Gait and balance training

Normal gait involves alternating states of single-leg stance with stepping. Single-leg stability is a very important component of gait and transfers for all ambulatory individuals. While the dynamic limb is moving, the stance leg is required to fully support the body, often experiencing greater challenges in stillness than the moving limb does in action. (Tub and car transfers require even longer periods of single-leg stance.) During single limb stability training, it is helpful for the stance leg to be maintained in slight knee flexion to facilitate balance reactions. The patient must be encouraged to contract the gluteus medius muscle to stabilize the stance hip and prevent a Trendelenburg reaction. Patients who can learn to coordinate a co-contraction of the abdominal and spinal muscles can be taught to maintain upright posture throughout a progression of more difficult drills.

Paterno, Myer, Ford, and Hewett (2004) conducted a study on the effects of neuromuscular training on single-leg stability in female athletes. The athletes participated in neuromuscular training 3x/week for 6 weeks. The training involved balance training and strengthening of the hip, pelvis, and trunk musculature. The authors concluded that single limb postural stability and proprioception are important components of lower extremity function and that a six-week neuromuscular training program can improve single limb postural stability.

Quick stepping in varying directions with fast stops provides a higher degree of challenge. A progression of speed requires faster balance reactions, including activation of stabilizing muscles. For example, moderate speed sidestepping requires fast activation of the peroneals to combat the lateral inertia. Good strength of the peroneals is important to ankle stability. If the peroneals are only trained at slow speeds in controlled environments, they may not be able to fire quickly in response to motion. This principle applies to all of the muscles involved in the stepping activities. Quick stopping is a large challenge, especially for knee patients. More specifically, ACL (anterior cruciate ligament)-deficient knees are challenged with quick stops on the involved knee. Quick stops involve a high degree of muscle co-contraction. In the absence of normal ligamentous support, the muscles must work even harder for dynamic control. Starting with slow steps forward onto the involved leg can allow the muscles to adjust to control the knee safely. Increasing the speed trains the muscles to respond more quickly.

Some examples of stance drills include:

Single leg static holds: This static activity is the foundational element for all single leg stability drills to follow. The core exercise involves balancing the body weight on one leg at a time and maintaining quiet stance. Perform this exercise with both eyes open; progress with both eyes closed for each leg. Stand on your left leg and raise your right foot off the ground. Flex (bend) your left knee slightly and hold that position for 2–3 seconds. Repeat with longer hold times. Repeat with the other leg.

Forward-backward swings (hip flexion/extension): In this variation, extension of the hip may provoke more co-contraction of the gastrocnemius/soleus and anterior tibialis muscles to stabilize the lower leg with the anterior/posterior motion. The patient is cued to maintain stance on one leg while moving the other leg first forwards and then backwards. Add repetitions as able to maintain balance on stance leg. The patient may be cued as follows: Stand straight with your right knee slightly bent. Raise your left leg behind

—— Proprioceptive Training ——

your body, keeping your knee straight. Tighten your abdominals slightly to control the position of your pelvis. Repeat with left leg.

Sideways swings (hip abduction): In this variation, the moving leg is focusing on gluteus medius muscle strengthening. The stance leg is also using the gluteus medius, but to control lateral stability, not to move. The patient must also activate the gluteus maximus and iliopsoas for hip extension/flexion control and the quadriceps and hamstrings for knee control. Specifically, hip abduction may require more peroneal muscle activation in the stance leg due to the lateral forces on the body. The patient can be cued as follows: Keep your body straight and your right knee slightly bent. Tighten your abdominals slightly to control the position of your pelvis. Raise your left leg out to the side, pause and slowly lower. Repeat with longer pauses or direction reversals. Repeat with the other leg.

Cross body leg swings: For performing this exercise, one needs to support oneself against a wall, facing it. Place your palms against the wall and stand slightly away from it. Swing your right leg towards the left, forward, as much as it can reach. Change leg and repeat the same with the left leg.

While some examples of steppage drills include:

Toe walking: This involves raising one's whole body on the toes and walking with the toes pointing ahead at first, then outwards and then inwards.

Heel walking: Bear weight on the heels keeping the toes up.

Step ups: Step ups are often used to target the quadriceps, but also strengthen the gluteus maximus and elicit co-contractions throughout the lower extremity muscles. Depending on the strength and functional level, the patient may start with step ups on 2-, 4- or 6-inch steps. UE support on parallel bars can be reduced from bilateral support to unilateral and possibly no UE support. Hold a railing or door frame as needed for support. Step up slowly on right leg and then lower. Repeat with left leg. Be sure that leg is in line with body.

Lunges: Lunges are used to strengthen the quadriceps and gluteus maximus as well as challenge the balance system throughout the body. With forward and lateral mini lunges, the person is moving the center of gravity and taking a large step. The size of the step and the speed of the motion determine the challenges and potential benefits of the exercise. The patient can face the parallel bars and do small lateral lunges. Step forward with the right leg and bend the knee while keeping the left knee nearly straight. Bring right leg back and do small lunges forward with left leg. Be sure that your body is upright, with shoulders over the hips. Repeat alternating legs. Then, step out to the right and bend the right knee. Your body weight should be shifting over your right leg with your trunk erect. Keep your left knee nearly straight. Bring right leg back to neutral and repeat with left leg.

Squats: Squats are used to strengthen the quadriceps and gluteus maximus as well as challenge the balance system throughout the body. Stand on right leg with left knee bent. Slowly bend right leg into a small squat and straighten. Repeat with left leg squats. The one leg squat is great not only for proprioception but also for stretching the quadriceps. One must be careful to not lunge forward. With greater familiarity, you can also hold dumbbells in hand when performing the one-leg squats.

Unstable surface drills

Walking on an uneven or giving surface provides additional training to the balance system. The foot and ankle complex is first to encounter an uneven surface. The body needs adequate proprioception to detect movements of the foot and ankle. When one walks on grass, the foot may invert and evert according to the uneven surface. Quick muscular responses to the changing foot position help to maintain balance and avoid an ankle sprain. If the balance reactions at the foot and ankle are inadequate or slow, then the person may lose overall balance and be at risk for a fall. If the rotational torque is not absorbed at the foot and ankle complex, excessive rotation may be transmitted to the knee joint. While the knee joint is capable of tibiofemoral rotation, large levels or fast speeds of rotation can stress the meniscus and even result in a meniscal tear. The rest of the body responds to the uneven surface.

McHugh, Tyler, Mirabella, Mullaney, and Nicholas (2007) followed two varsity football teams for three seasons and found that single-limb balance training on a foam stability pad reduced the injury incidence by 77%, eliminating the risk of ankle sprain associated with a previous ankle sprain and/or a high body mass index (BMI). The balance training in this study was done for five minutes on each leg, five days a week for four weeks in preseason, then two times a week for nine weeks during the season. McHugh et al. (2007) did not find any effect on injury incidence with taping or brace use. Therefore, this study found only single-limb balance training to be effective in reducing the risk of ankle sprain in football players.

—— Proprioceptive Training ——

Mohammadi (2007) conducted a study on 80 male soccer players with a history of inversion sprain. Group one focused on proprioceptive training with an ankle disc, standing on the involved leg and shifting weight for circular motion of the disc with a progression from eyes open to closed, firm to soft surfaces. Group two had focused strengthening of the evertor muscles with a progression from isometric to dynamic and then resistive exercise. Group three had an Air cast brace and Group four did not have any intervention. Mohammadi (2007) concluded that proprioceptive training was more effective in reducing the rate of ankle sprains than no intervention. Interestingly, no significant injury rate reduction was found with the strengthening or Air cast groups. Ankle proprioceptive deficits may result in slow activation of the muscles, especially the evertors, with a failure to correct excessive ankle positions. Wester, Jespersen, Nielsen, and Neumann (1996) studied wobble board training after primary Stage 2 ankle sprains and found that it was effective in reducing residual symptoms but that it did not affect the time course of edema reduction.

Some examples of unstable surface drills include:

Rocker board, wobble board or biomechanical ankle platform system (BAPS) balance board drills

Place feet shoulder-width apart on the rocker board (or other device) and rock side to side. Then turn the board forward and rock forward and backward. Keep the knees slightly bent and the trunk erect. After rocking side to side, try to balance in the middle with knees slightly bent. Add arm raises for changes to the center of gravity. Turn the rocker board to a forward position and repeat. Practice ball toss on rocker board. Vary toss direction and speed. Place desired ball size on underside of BAPS to create target balance exercise. Stand on involved leg with foot in marked position. Roll foot in circular motion. Then, stand and attempt to balance in one position.

Foam pad or BOSU Pro Balance Trainer exercises

Stand on BOSU Pro Balance Trainer (or a foam pad) to challenge standing balance. Then, slowly squat on BOSU Pro Balance Trainer. To progress, increase depth of squat as able. Do mini forward and lateral lunges and land with lunge leg onto BOSU Pro Balance Trainer. Try standing hip flexion, extension, and abduction on BOSU Pro Balance Trainer. You can also try single-leg squats on BOSU Pro Balance Trainer. Do ball catch on BOSU Pro Balance Trainer. Vary speed and direction of ball as tolerated.

Trampoline exercises

Stand in middle of trampoline with feet shoulder-width apart. Do squats to 45–60° knee flexion. Then, do standing hip abduction on trampoline. Start with one movement per repetition and progress to a series of hip abduction movements per repetition. This increases the balance challenge by increasing the time in single-leg stance. Repeat with standing hip flexion and extension. Play catch with the patient while he or she is on a trampoline. Vary the ball tosses high and low and side to side.

Plyometrics and agility training

Plyometrics and agility training are often included in late-stage rehabilitation. Myer et al. (2006) used a comprehensive program of resistance training for upper extremity, lower extremity, and core muscles as well as speed interval training and cut maneuvers in single and double-leg stance. The first treatment group added plyometric training, with frequent feedback for technical performance of jumping and cutting. The second group added balance and stability exercises instead of the plyometric exercises. All programs were done 3x/week for 7 weeks for 90 minutes each session. The balance and dynamic stability exercises included dynamic lower extremity stabilization and balance exercises in single and double stance. The athletes were instructed on methods to dampen landing force through sagittal plane flexion with avoidance of knee valgus. In this study, Myer et al. (2006) found both the plyometric and the balance training programs were effective in decreasing factors related to ACL injury and increasing performance. The balance group had a larger improvement in single limb force attenuation strategies.

With jumping training, the focus is on equalizing ground reaction force attenuation strategies (Myer et al., 2006). Thighs should be parallel to the floor with starting and landing shoulder-width apart. There should be symmetry on takeoff, in air, and upon landing. The clinician may also include single limb hops for distance, vertical power hops, and lateral hops. The athlete must increase confidence and stability with high intensity changes of directional activities. A crucial form factor is safe biomechanics with increased knee flexion and decreased knee abduction angles with high-level plyometric activities (Myer et al. 2006).

Lloyd (2001) reported that training to reduce muscle voluntary reaction time is beneficial since quick directional changes increase varus-valgus and internal-external rotation loading of the knee. Reaction time is also crucial at the foot and ankle level to avoid an ankle sprain. Jumping and hopping are popular components of rehabilitation training that often emphasize the plyometric aspect. Hopping is best started with landing on both feet for maximal stability and control. As the athlete progresses, he may start unilateral landing. It is ideal to start single-leg landings on the uninvolved leg for training purposes. Then the athlete may start hopping onto the involved leg. The directions of the hops may be varied to challenge the muscles with co-contraction and stabilization in varied positions and directions. Hopping is a predominant feature of late-stage sport training for ACL reconstruction patients and hopping forward imposes a large strain on the ACL of the landing leg and must be approved by the surgeon.

In addition to power concerns, jumping training is important for landing control. Landing training may be done as the athlete jumps off of an 8" or 10" step while the clinician monitors ankle and knee stability. In addition, it is good to train the athlete to land softly with some degree of knee flexion. A small degree of knee flexion on landing facilitates co-contraction of the quadriceps and hamstrings to help protect the knee. Do all exercises with feet shoulder-width apart. Be sure to land with knees bent with good landing form with knees in line with lower legs.

Some examples of jump and agility training include:

> *Basic jump:* do quick squat and jump up and land softly with knees bent. Then, do a quick squat and hop to the side. Place tape strips on the floor as targets for lateral hops. Then, do a quick squat and hop forward across the room.

> *Step jump:* Start with left foot on box with knee bent and right foot on floor. Do quick squat and jump up and over the box, landing on the other side of the step up box with the right foot on the box and left foot on the floor. You can also jump forward off a step up box. Repeat in opposite direction.

> *Obstacle hops:* Do quick repetitive hops in zigzag pattern over small cones.

> *Alternating side jump:* Do a lateral jump to the right side and land on the right leg. Stay slightly on toes throughout the exercise. Be sure that the right knee is slightly bent at landing. Then jump to the left and land on the left leg with the left knee slightly bent.

> *Alternating forward jump*: Do a forward jump onto the right leg and land with right knee slightly bent. Repeat with the left leg.

> *Braiding run:* Do a cross-over run laterally, placing left foot in front of right leg. Then cross over left foot behind left leg and bring right leg out to the side. Do cross over run to the right and then back to the left.

> *Squat drills:* Maintain a small squat position on toes with knees bent. Do forward and backward hops landing onto both feet. Do lateral hops onto both feet. Do mini forward, backward, and lateral mini runs. Stay in a mini squat position.

—— *Proprioceptive Training* ——

Mind-body therapies

Yoga

Yoga has long been practiced as a method for physical training in India. Yoga techniques that deal with increasing physical strength and flexibility have been described in ancient as well as modern Indian literature. Yoga exercises also include a component of regulated breathing (pranayama). Yoga as a health restorative practice has been adopted by people in various cultures. In ancient Indian scriptures yoga was described as a practice that initiates and establishes physical well-being in the first phase, helps the individual to attain conscious 'control' over the five senses of the body in the next stage, and helps the individual attain spiritual enlightenment in the final stage. Belief in the spiritual benefits of any practice is a subjective matter and quite beyond the scope of the present discussion.

The benefits of yoga in restoring and maintaining physical well-being cannot be ignored.

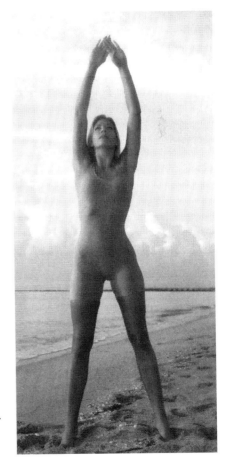

In a study conducted by Hart and Tracy (2008), young adult participants (n=10, 29 +/- 6 years) were asked to perform standard yoga exercises for 24 sessions lasting eight weeks. Each session lasted for an hour and a half wherein the subjects were asked to perform standard yoga poses under supervision.

The control group consisted of age-matched young adults (n=11, 26 +/- 7 years) who were not exposed to yoga exercises. Hart and Tracy (2008) monitored the maximum voluntary contraction force (MVC) on the elbow flexor and knee extensor muscles, steadiness of isometric contractions of these muscles, steadiness of concentric and eccentric contractions of knee extensors, and timed balance for each of the participants.

Participants who underwent yoga training demonstrated a 14% increase in the maximum voluntary contraction force with the knee extensors. The training did not have any discernible effect on the elbow flexor muscles. Concentric and eccentric contractions in the

—— Proprioceptive Training ——

knee extensor muscles were also largely unaffected in terms of force exerted. However, the steadiness of these contractions was increased. People who showed the least steadiness in the contraction measurements with knee extensors showed reduced variations following yoga training. The timed balance measurements showed that yoga participants had greater balance as compared to the control group.

Yoga exercises seem to improve the balance and steadiness in people who seem to be inherently unsteady. Although the yoga training resulted in a modest increase in strength, the important outcomes were greater muscle control, reduction in involuntary contractions, and enhanced balance. Yoga may have a role to play in reduction of injuries in people since increase in inherent stability can be correlated with reduction in injuries (McGuine et al., 2000; McGuine & Keene 2006).

Yoga was also shown to be effective in improving gait in elderly people (Telles et al., 1993). In a study group, 69 elderly individuals aged 60 to 95 were randomly assigned to three groups. One group received yoga training, the other was treated with an herbal Ayurvedic medicine (which is supposed to increase muscle strength), and the third was the control group with no exercise and treatment. The control group, however, observed the normal behavioral activities like reading watching TV and playing indoor games. The average age of participants in each group was 71 years.

In this study, yoga sessions were conducted for 75 minutes every day. These sessions included loosening (stretching) exercises for 5 minutes; breathing exercises for 10 minutes; physical postures (aka asanas) for 20 minutes; voluntarily regulated breathing (pranayama) for 10 minutes; yoga-based guided relaxation for 15 minutes; and devotional songs (bhajans) for 15 minutes.

Baseline measurements for gait, balance, and mobility were recorded using the Tinetti Balance and Gait Evaluation Test as well as the timed up and go test (TUG). In the TUG test, participants seated in a chair placed three meters from a wall were asked to rise and walk to the wall, turn around, walk back, and be seated again. The number of walking steps taken to perform this task was measured; a lower score indicated higher limb function. All the participants were assessed for changes in gait, balance, and mobility on the same criteria after six months of the respective intervention.

At the end of six months, the yoga group showed significant improvements in gait ($p<0.001$) and balance ($p<0.01$) over baseline measurements. The other two groups did not show any improvement over their baseline measurements. In the mobility tests, both the Ayurvedic potion group and yoga group showed significant improvement. Yoga exercises proved to be beneficial both by increasing proprioception as well as improving muscle strength. Consumption of the ayurvedic medicinal preparation could have also resulted in improved muscle strength leading to lower scores on the TUG test. However, since gait is the net result of movement of limbs, dynamic balance, and visual perception, these results clearly indicate proprioceptive benefits of yoga. The fact that improvements were seen in elderly patients is also very important.

It is important to note, though, that people of age 60 and above are not capable of performing physically challenging exercise routines like treadmill sessions or work with balance boards and resistance bands. Sometimes even mundane daily physical activities can seem like insurmountable challenges to them. And yet, in this study, not only was the group of septuagenarians successful in following yoga postures, but they were also able to derive neuromuscular facilitation from them. These results emphasize the proprioceptive benefits of yoga. More studies investigating the role of yoga as a rehabilitative technique are certainly warranted; however, the potential to use this ancient Indian practice is surely indicated.

T'ai Chi-Qigong (T'ai Chi)

T'ai Chi-Qigong, or T'ai Chi as it is more popularly known, is an ancient Chinese exercise form designed to enhance balance and muscle tension regulation. Although the health benefits derived from practicing T'ai Chi have been accepted in Chinese cultures, the specific effects of T'ai Chi on biomechanics have not been studied in detail.

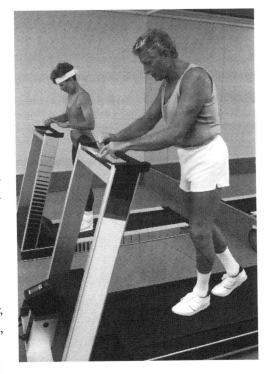

In order to understand the effects of T'ai Chi exercises and Qigong meditation, a controlled clinical trial was conducted by Yang et al. in 2007. In this randomized controlled trial, 33 healthy octogenarians were trained in T'ai Chi exercises coupled with Qigong mediation. Sixteen age-matched individuals served as age-matched controls. T'ai Chi-Qigong was practiced by the experimental group for one hour per session with three sessions per week for a total period of six months. The Sensory Organization Test was applied to estimate somatosensory, visual and vestibular inputs. Likewise, the quiet stance Base of Support (BoS) and opening of feet angle tests were used to assess balance in the participants. These measurements were conducted prior to the intervention (T0), at two months (T2), and six months into the trial (T6) time points.

Reference: Broglio SP, Ferrara MS, Sopiarz K, Kelly MS. Reliable change of the sensory organization test. Clin J Sport Med. 2008 Mar;18(2):148-54. doi: 10.1097/ JSM.0b013e318164f42a.

Sensory Organization Test

Purpose: Sensory organization test is a form of posturography which is designed to assess quantitatively an individual's ability to use visual, proprioceptive and vestibular cues to maintain postural stability in stance.

Description: Subjects stand on dual-force plates in a 3-sided surround. The anterior-posterior sway is recorded.

There are 6 independent sensory conditions tested, each condition consisting of three twenty second trials:

The conditions are:

1. Eyes open on firm surface,
2. Eyes closed on firm surface
3. Eyes open with sway referenced visual surround,
4. Eyes open on sway referenced support surface,
5. Eyes closed on sway referenced support surface,
6. Eyes open on sway referenced support surface and surround

The outcome measures are:

1. Equilibrium Score, which is the average center of gravity, sway for each trial for each condition
2. The composite equilibrium score, which is a weighted average of the six conditions. It is derived from the individual equilibrium scores
3. The sensory analysis ratios, which are computed averages to identify impairments of individual sensory systems.
4. Center of gravity (COG) Alignment which reflects the patient's COG position relative to the center of the base of support at the start of each trial of the SOT
5. Strategy Analysis quantifies the relative amount of movement about the ankles (ankle strategy) and about the hips (hip strategy) the patient used to maintain balance during each trial.

Proprioceptive Training

The findings showed that the T'ai Chi-Qigong group showed increased vestibular contribution to the sensory organization test at T2 (22% increase over that at T0) and T6 (47 % increase over that at T0). The participants also showed better quiet stance in the BoS test but no changes in the foot angle opening metrics. T'ai Chi-Qigong techniques therefore seem to enhance vestibular inputs, thereby increasing balance and steadiness in people who practice these techniques. Similar results have also been reported by Tsang and Hui-Chan (2004) in a trial with elderly participants.

In both these studies, short T'ai Chi routines were taught to the participants instead of lengthy and continuously executed choreography. Yet the proprioceptive effects of T'ai Chi have been apparent very early into the training program, at four weeks in the Tsang and Hui-Chan study (2004) and at eight weeks in the work described by Yang et al. (2007).

In another study, T'ai Chi training helped to improve knee extensor muscle strength as well as force control (Christou, Yang, & Rosengren, 2003). In this study, a cohort of 16 septuagenarians was trained in T'ai Chi for 20 weeks prior to assessment. Ten elderly people of mean age 74 years were included in the control group. Following the 20-week period of T'ai Chi training, there was a 19.5 % increase in the maximum voluntary contraction of the knee extensor muscles. The participants also simultaneously showed a decrease in the coefficient of variations in the isometric knee extension tasks, suggesting enhanced ability to control muscular behavior (Christou et al., 2003).

Taken together, results of these trials are very important in geriatric health. Prevention of injuries is a huge concern in maintaining health in geriatric citizens. Elderly citizens are also prone to falls due to loss of balance with age. Elderly people, even those who are free from other systemic diseases, have difficulty healing bone fractures. Prevention of falls and imbalance injuries seems to be the best strategy to avoid serious health impairments in elderly people. Hence, restorative therapies that enhance balance and restore muscle strength enough to confer independent mobility are essential for geriatric citizens.

In this respect, yoga and T'ai Chi (T'ai Chi) are very significant proprioceptive training techniques that can serve to maintain strength in lower extremities in even septuagenarians. The important thing is that in both systems of exercise, short training periods seem to show a rapid and favorable outcome in neuromuscular facilitation. Also, the training techniques can be adapted to suit the strength level of old people, which may not always be the case with equipment-assisted therapy.

T'ai Chi and Yoga also include a psychological healing touch in the form of Qigong meditation and Pranayama and spiritual components, respectively. These facets are also important in helping older citizens in overcoming the trauma of the accidents experienced by them. The psychological solace imparted by these techniques may also prove to be valuable in allowing the patient to heal and regain physical capability.

Aquatic therapy

Aquatic therapy and exercise in water is a relative newcomer to the rehabilitation arena. The polio outbreaks around the time of World War I were perhaps the catalysts for the worldwide dissemination of aquatic therapy as a viable treatment option. The revolutionary ideas to move rather than immobilize paralyzed limbs, led to an increased attention to the difficulties that land-based therapeutic exercise posed for those with proprioceptive and movement deficits; the swimming pool became an attractive venue for treatment. Over the last century, aquatic therapy has changed drastically and there are now highly evolved specialty techniques, which are performed solely in water. The most popular of these techniques are described here.

Ai Chi

Ai Chi is a water-based strengthening program and a form of active relaxation, which seeks to integrate physical, mental and spiritual energy. It has analogies with Watsu, but also uses the techniques of Qi Gong and Tai Chi Chuan to enhance the flow of life energy (Chinese qi) through movement-based stimulation of meridian acupoints. It is performed standing in water, and begins with breathing exercises and progresses to 19 katas, broad and slow movements of the extremities and trunk that are accomplished without force at the rate of breathing. These movements stretch the lung meridian by retracting the scapula, the small intestine meridian by scapular protraction, the bladder meridian through opening of the sacroiliac joint, and extension of the thoracic and lumbar spine to affect the kidney meridian. It has been shown to enhance strength and range of motion, and also increases oxygen consumption and calorie expenditure. Reduced stress and increased alertness have been reported, and Eastern practitioners believe the technique improves blood circulation and decreases liver stagnation while Western therapists suggest that it improves kinesthetic sense and therefore coordination as well as creating "design sense", the feeling of doing what the body was designed to do. It has therefore been advocated for chronic and especially painful conditions as well as respiratory, cardiac and psychological disorders and problems of overeating and obesity (Lambeck and Bommer, 1997).

The largest and most comprehensive randomized controlled trial of the effectiveness of Ai Chi was reported by Castro Sanchez et al. (2012). Ai Chi aquatic exercise was compared with abdominal breathing and contraction-relaxation exercises, and the effect of treatment on pain, depression, fatigue, spasticity and functional independence was assessed before and after treatment and at 4 and 10 weeks of therapy in 73 patients with multiple sclerosis. Pain was assessed by Visual Analog Scale and Pain Rating Index, along with the Present Pain Intensity scale of the McGill Pain Questionnaire. Depression was quantified with the Beck Depression Inventory, fatigue by the Modified Fatigue Impact Scale, and spasticity by Visual Analog and Multiple Sclerosis Impact Scales. The Roland Morris Disability Questionnaire and Barthel Index of Activities of Daily Living. Ai Chi was carried out in 36°C water and land-based exercises at 26°C during 60-minute sessions. Pain intensity was significantly decreased with aquatic exercise, while spasticity, fatigue, and degree of disability were significantly lessened and level of autonomy significantly increased. The control patients did not show improvement in these parameters. The improvements were ascribed to amelioration of fatigue, lessening of depression and less impairment by spasticity during water exercise; background music, which promotes rhythmic movement in water and may affect the oscillations of brain circadian timekeepers was also suggested as a contributory factor, as the aquatic exercise was performed with background music and the control exercise was not.

Bad Ragaz Ring Method

The **Bad Ragaz Ring Method** exercises utilize several beneficial properties of water: buoyancy, turbulence, surface tension and thermal capacity. Its goals are muscle re-education, strengthening, relaxation, tone reduction or inhibition and application of spinal traction when necessary. Initially, range-of-motion exercises were performed on treatment boards fixed in the water, with the body secured by straps or anchored by rails on the side of the pool. Knupfer and Ipsen modified this to support the client by flotation rings under the knees and ankles and around the neck and pelvis during active resistance exercises. Active movements away from and back to the fixed point of the therapist's hands allowed closed kinetic chain exercise in the supportive medium of water, with additional physiological benefits from warm water. Three-dimensional diagonal movements effective for reducing spasticity were subsequently imported from proprioceptive neuromuscular facilitation. The technique allows for isokinetic exercise, in which the therapist provides fixation and the client moves away from, toward or around the therapist, the speed of the client's movements determining the resistance. The therapist can also be a "movable" point of fixation in isotonic exercise, increasing resistance by pushing or swinging the client in the direction of movement, or can isometrically push the client in a fixed position through the water, thereby promoting stabilization. Benefits may include reduced tone, relaxation, increased range of motion, muscle re-education, increased strength, spinal traction, preparation of the

—— Proprioceptive Training ——

lower extremities for weight bearing, greater stability of the trunk and increased endurance (Garrett, 1997).

Halliwick Method

The **Halliwick method** is aimed at the "core stabilization", which is the achievement of postural control, necessary in the horizontal for swimming but important in the vertical for standing and walking. Independence is its goal, which requires the willingness to lose one's balance if necessary and the ability to regain it if lost. Moving water provides impedance, so balance will be lost slowly and there is time to react. The force of gravity is counteracted by the buoyancy of water, and rotation in the water causes torque, which can increase load on connective tissues with strengthening effect. Position can be changed more easily in a buoyant medium, which influences the vestibular system and facilitates sensory integration, so the method is potentially useful for those with disturbed equilibrium. A graded activity program with low impact is possible in an environment of reduced gravity, which should be helpful in the setting of hemiparesis or hemiplegia (Cunningham, 1997).

Noh, Lim, Shin and Paik (2008) assessed the effects of aquatic therapy on 13 ambulatory stroke rehabilitation patients to 12 receiving conventional physical therapy. Both groups had 3 one-hour sessions a week for 8 weeks, and the experimental group took part in Ai Chi and Halliwick exercises. The Berg Balance Score and vertical ground reaction force during standing tasks were measured, along with manual muscle testing and gait speed. Standing tasks involved rising from a chair and then shifting weight forward, backward and laterally. The Ai Chi and Halliwick participants had significantly improved Berg Balance Scores, forward and backward weight- bearing and knee flexor strength as compared to patients who performed aerobic exercises. The study, again a small sample treated for a relatively short time, suggested that the swimming-based therapies are effective for improving balance and postural control.

Aquatic therapy was studied in the first weeks of inpatient stroke rehabilitation by Tripp and Krakow (2013). Thirty patients who were hospitalized after first-ever stroke 2 weeks or more previously had either Halliwick aquatic therapy for 45 minutes three times a week or conventional physiotherapy five times weekly. Postural stability as measured by the Berg Balance Scale and functional reach, functional gait and functional mobility measures were compared before and after 2 weeks of treatment. Significant improvement in the Berg Balance Scale occurred in 83.3 percent of the Halliwick therapy group *versus* 46.7 percent of the conventional physiotherapy group. The Halliwick therapy patients were significantly more improved in functional gait ability, but the other measures did not show a significant difference in improvement between the groups. This study suggests that Halliwick aquatic therapy can improve balance and gait after stroke, and that it might be effective in the immediate post-stroke rehabilitative period.

Watsu

Watsu is passive aquatic bodywork that involves slow movements in water to induce relaxation and to enhance the parasympathetic and quiet the sympathetic nervous system. The method derives from the stretching movements of Zen Shiatsu, which are thought to open the channels through which universal energy ("ki" in Japanese) flows. Stretching also increases muscle flexibility and diminishes nerve compression and resultant somatic dysfunction. Connection with the breath and elements of dance while floating add a meditative component. Heart rate, respiratory rate and skeletal muscle tone are reduced, while depth of respiration; smooth muscle activity, peripheral vasodilatation and immune function are increased. Range of motion is increased and spasticity or pain decreased in the short term, and reported long-term benefits involve sleep, digestion, healing and immunocompetence and control of pain and anxiety. (Dull, 1997).

Chon, Oh and Shim (2009) assessed the effect of the Watsu method on spasticity and balance in 3 hemiparetic stroke patients. Watsu sessions were given 5 times a week for 8 weeks, and the Rivermead Visual Gait Assessment and Tone Assessment Scale were carried out before and after the 40 treatments. The patients showed significant improvement in spastic gait, imbalance on walking and abnormal muscle tone with Watsu, but their small number limits generalization of the result.

Conclusion

There may be no magic formula in providing the "perfect" proprioceptive challenge for any patient. Almost any of the exercises typically used in physical therapy can have a dynamic element introduced integrated and thus become a proprioceptive task. For instance, squats and lunges can be performed onto a BOSU ball. Single limb stance can be progressed by adding head turns, changes in position of the contralateral leg, arm swings, closing eyes, or by adding a cognitive task, such as counting backwards by 3's. Ambulation can be progressed by adding an elastic band to the ankle and performing "figure-8" walks. Strength training can be moved from the mat to the Pilates Reformer for a more dynamic effect. The important consideration is whether or not the patient is being challenged beyond current boundaries and made to attempt novel scenarios. This is the heart and soul of proprioceptive rehabilitation.

REFERENCES

Abbruzzese, G., Trompetto, C., Mori, L., & Pelosin, E. (2014). Proprioceptive rehabilitation of upper limb dysfunction in movement disorders: a clinical perspective. *Frontiers in human neuroscience*, *8*.

Ackerman, D. B., Trousdale, R. T., Bieber, P., Henely, J., Pagnano, M. W., & Berry, D. J. (2010). Postoperative patient falls on an orthopedic inpatient unit. *The Journal of Arthroplasty*, *25*(1), 10-14. http://www.ncbi.nlm.nih.gov/pubmed/19062249

American College of Foot and Ankle Surgeons (3/2/12). Ankle Replacement Rapidly on the Rise. Retrieved from http://www.acfas.org/content.aspx?id=2971.

American Geriatrics Society, British Geriatrics Society, American Academy of Orthopaedic Surgeons. Guideline for the prevention of falls in older persons. American Geriatrics Society, British Geriatrics Society, and American Academy of Orthopaedic Surgeons Panel on Falls Prevention. J Am Geriatr Soc. 2001;49:664–72.

Arkin, S. (2007). Language-enriched exercise plus socialization slows cognitive decline in Alzheimer's disease. *American journal of Alzheimer's disease and other dementias*, *22*(1), 62–77.

Arkin, S. M. (1999). Elder rehabilitation: A student-supervised exercise program for Alzheimer's patients. *The Gerontologist*, *39*(6), 729–35.

Arkin, S. M. (2003). Student-led exercise sessions yield significant fitness gains for Alzheimer's patients. *American journal of Alzheimer's disease and other dementias*, *18*(3), 159–70.

Arnold, S. A., Stewart, A. M., Moor, H. M., Karl, R. C., & Reneker, J. C. (2015). The Effectiveness of Vestibular Rehabilitation Interventions in Treating Unilateral Peripheral Vestibular Disorders: A Systematic Review. Physiotherapy Research International.

Assaiante, C. (1998). Development of locomotor balance control in healthy children. *Neuroscience and biobehavioral reviews, 22*(4), 527–32.

Badke M. B., Sherman J., Boyne P., Page S., Dunning K. (2011). Tongue-based biofeedback for balance in stroke: results of an 8-week pilot study. Arch. Phys. Med. Rehabil. 92, 1364–1370. 10.1016/j.apmr.2011.03.030

Bakan P., Thompson R. W. (1967). Induction and retention of kinesthetic aftereffects as a function of number and distribution of inspection trials. Percept. Psychophys. 2, 304–306 10.3758/BF03211047

Barbar, A., Bahadoran, R., Ghasemzadeh, Y. The effect of aquatic exercise on balance of adults with multiple sclerosis. European Journal of Experimental Biology, 2014;4(1):38-43.

Beets I. A. M., Macé M., Meesen R. L. J., Cuypers K., Levin O., Swinnen S. P. (2012). Active versus passive training of a complex bimanual task: is prescriptive proprioceptive information sufficient for inducing motor learning? PLoS ONE 7:e37687. 10.1371/journal.pone.0037687

Berger, W.,Trippel, M., Assainte, C., Zijlstra, W., Dietz, V. (1995) Developmental aspects of equilibrium control during stance: a kinematic and EMG study. Gait Posture 3:149–155.

Bosco, G., & Poppele, R. E. (2001). Proprioception from a spinocerebellar perspective. *Physiological reviews, 81*(2), 539–68.

Bressel, E., Yonker, J. C., Kras, J., & Heath, E. M. (2007). Comparison of static and dynamic balance in female collegiate soccer, basketball, and gymnastics athletes. *Journal of Athletic Training, 42*(1), 42–6.

Bronson C, Brewerton K, Ong J, Palanca C, Sullivan SJ. Does hippotherapy improve balance in persons with multiple sclerosis: a systematic review. European journal of physical and rehabilitation medicine. Sep 2010;46(3):347-353

Buchman, A. S., Wilson, R. S., & Bennett, D. A. (2008). Total daily activity is associated with cognition in older persons. *The American journal of geriatric psychiatry : official journal of the American Association for Geriatric Psychiatry, 16*,(8), 697–701. Doi: 10.1097/JGP.0b013e31817945f6

Cameron MH, Lord S. Postural control in multiple sclerosis: implications for fall prevention. Current neurology and neuroscience reports. Sep 2010;10(5):407-412.

Carel C., Loubinoux I., Boulanouar K., Manelfe C., Rascol O., Celsis P., et al. . (2000). Neural substrate for the effects of passive training on sensorimotor cortical representation:

a study with functional magnetic resonance imaging in healthy subjects. J. Cereb. Blood Flow Metab. 20, 478–484. 10.1097/00004647-200003000-00006

Carey L. M., Matyas T. A. (2005). Training of somatosensory discrimination after stroke. Am. J. Phys. Med. Rehabil. 84, 428–442. 10.1097/01.PHM.0000159971.12096.7F

Carey L. M., Matyas T. A., Oke L. E. (1993). Sensory loss in stroke patients: effective training of tactile and proprioceptive discrimination. Arch. Phys. Med. Rehabil. 74, 602–611. 10.1016/0003-9993(93)90158-7

Casadio M., Giannoni P., Morasso P., Sanguineti V. (2009a). A proof of concept study for the integration of robot therapy with physiotherapy in the treatment of stroke patients. Clin. Rehabil. 23, 217–228. 10.1177/0269215508096759

Casadio M., Morasso P., Sanguineti V., Giannoni P. (2009b). Minimally assistive robot training for proprioception enhancement. Exp. Brain Res. 194, 219–231. 10.1007/s00221-008-1680-6

Case-Smith J., Weaver L., & Fristad M. (2014). A systematic review of sensory processing interventions for children with autism spectrum disorders. *Autism.*

CDC - Arthritis - Basics - Definition - Rheumatoid Arthritis. (Updated November 6, 2014). Retrieved from http://www.cdc.gov/arthritis/basics/rheumatoid.htm

Chen J. C., Lin C. H., Wei Y. C., Hsiao J., Liang C. C. (2011). Facilitation of motor and balance recovery by thermal intervention for the paretic lower limb of acute stroke: a single-blind randomized clinical trial. Clin. Rehabil. 25, 823–832. 10.1177/0269215511399591

Chinnavan, E., Gopaladhas, S., Saha, A., & Ragupathy, R. (2014). Effectiveness of Proprioceptive Training in Grade-ii Acute Anterior Cruciate Ligament Injury in Athletes. Indian Journal of Science and Technology, 7(12), 2041-2045.

Chouza M., Arias P., Vinas S., Cudeiro J. (2011). Acute effects of whole-body vibration at 3, 6, and 9 hz on balance and gait in patients with Parkinson's disease. Mov. Disord. 26, 920–921. 10.1002/mds.23582

Christou, E. A., Yang, Y., & Rosengren, K. S. (2003). Taiji training improves knee extensor strength and force control in older adults. *The journals of gerontology Series A Biological sciences and medical sciences*, 58(8), 763–6.

Conrad M. O., Scheidt R. A., Schmit B. D. (2011). Effects of wrist tendon vibration on arm tracking in people poststroke. J. Neurophysiol. 106, 1480–1488. 10.1152/jn.00404.2010

Cordo P., Lutsep H., Cordo L., Wright W. G., Cacciatore T., Skoss R. (2009). Assisted movement with enhanced sensation (AMES): coupling motor and sensory to remediate motor deficits in chronic stroke patients. Neurorehabil. Neural Repair 23, 67–77. 10.1177/1545968308317437

Cumpston, A. & Coles, A. (2008). Multiple Sclerosis. Lancet, 372(9648): 1502-1517.

de Oliveira R., Cacho E. W., Borges G. (2007). Improvements in the upper limb of hemiparetic patients after reaching movements training. Int. J. Rehabil. Res. 30, 67–70. 10.1097/MRR.0b013e3280143bbf

Dechaumont-Palacin S., Marque P., De Boissezon X., Castel-Lacanal E., Carel C., Berry I., et al. . (2008). Neural correlates of proprioceptive integration in the contralesional hemisphere of very impaired patients shortly after a subcortical stroke: an FMRI study. Neurorehabil. Neural Repair 22, 154–165. 10.1177/1545968307307118

Di Rienzo, F., Collet, C., Hoyek, N., & Guillot, A. (2014). Impact of neurologic deficits on motor imagery: a systematic review of clinical evaluations. Neuropsychology review, 24(2), 116-147.

Diracoglu D., Aydin R., Baskent A., Celik A. (2005). Effects of kinesthesia and balance exercises in knee osteoarthritis. J. Clin. Rheumatol. 11, 303–310.

Ebersbach G., Edler D., Kaufhold O., Wissel J. (2008). Whole body vibration versus conventional physiotherapy to improve balance and gait in Parkinson's disease. Arch. Phys. Med. Rehabil. 89, 399–403. 10.1016/j.apmr.2007.09.031

Eggermont, L., Swaab, D., Luiten, P., & Scherder, E. (2006). Exercise, cognition and Alzheimer's disease: More is not necessarily better. *Neuroscience and biobehavioral reviews*, *30*(4), 562–75. Doi: 10.1016/j.neubiorev.2005.10.004

Eils E., Rosenbaum D. (2001). A multi-station proprioceptive exercise program in patients with ankle instability. Med. Sci. Sports Exerc. 33, 1991–1998. 10.1097/00005768-200112000-00003

Eils E., Schroter R., Schroder M., Gerss J., Rosenbaum D. (2010). Multistation proprioceptive exercise program prevents ankle injuries in basketball. Med. Sci. Sports Exerc. 42, 2098–2105. 10.1249/MSS.0b013e3181e03667

Fisher, B. E., Wu, A.D., Salem, G. J., Song, J., & Lin, C. H. (2008). The effect of exercise training in improving motor performance and corticomotor excitability in people with early Parkinson's disease. *Archives of physical medicine and rehabilitation, 89*(7), 1221–9. Doi: 10.1016/j.apmr.2008.01.013

Fu, A. S., & Hui-Chan, C. W. (2005). Ankle joint proprioception and postural control in basketball players with bilateral ankle sprains. *The American journal of sports medicine, 33*(8), 1174–82.

Ganesan, M., Sathyaprabha, T. N., Gupta, A., & Pal, P. K. (2014). Effect of Partial Weight–Supported Treadmill Gait Training on Balance in Patients With Parkinson Disease. PM&R, 6(1), 22-33.

Gatti, R., Tettamanti, A., Gough, P. M., Riboldi, E., Marinoni, L., & Buccino, G. (2013). Action observation versus motor imagery in learning a complex motor task: a short review of literature and a kinematics study. Neuroscience Letters, 540, 37-42.

Goodwin, V. A., Richards, S. H., Taylor, R. S., Taylor, A. H., & Campbell, J. L. (2008). The effectiveness of exercise interventions for people with Parkinson's disease: A systematic review and meta- analysis. *Movement disorders : official journal of the Movement Disorder Society, 23*(5), 631–40. Doi: 10.1002/mds.21922

González-Ortega, D., Díaz-Pernas, F. J., Martínez-Zarzuela, M., & Antón-Rodríguez, M. (2014). A Kinect-based system for cognitive rehabilitation exercises monitoring. Computer methods and programs in biomedicine, 113(2), 620-631.

Gougoulias, N. E., Khanna, A., & Maffulli, N. (2009). History and evolution in total ankle arthroplasty. British Medical Bulletin, 89(1), 111–51. doi:10.1093/bmb/ldn039

Grampurohit, N., Pradhan, S., & Kartin, D. (2015). Efficacy of adhesive taping as an adjunt to physical rehabilitation to influence outcomes post-stroke: a systematic review. *Topics in stroke rehabilitation, 22*(1), 72-82.

Gstoettner, M., Raschner, C., Dirnberger, E., Leimser, H., & Krismer, M. (2011). Preoperative proprioceptive training in patients with total knee arthroplasty. The Knee, 18(4), 265-270.

Gurley, J. M., Hujsak, B. D., & Kelly, J. L. (2013). Vestibular rehabilitation following mild traumatic brain injury. NeuroRehabilitation, 32(3), 519-528. Haas C. T., Buhlmann A., Turbanski S., Schmidtbleicher D. (2006). Proprioceptive and sensorimotor performance in Parkinson's disease. Res. Sports Med. 14, 273–287. 10.1080/15438620600985902

Hart, C. E., & Tracy, B. L. (2008). Yoga as steadiness training: Effects on motor variability in young adults. *Journal of strength and conditioning research / National Strength & Conditioning Association*, *22*(5), 1659–69. Doi: 10.1519/JSC.0b013e31818200dd

Heremans, E., Nieuwboer, A., Feys, P., Vercruysse, S., Vandenberghe, W., Sharma, N., & Helsen, W. F. (2012). External cueing improves motor imagery quality in patients with Parkinson disease. *Neurorehabilitation and neural repair*, *26*(1), 27-35.Herz, N. B., Mehta, S. H., Sethi, K. D., Jackson, P., Hall, P., & Morgan, J. C. (2013). Nintendo Wii rehabilitation ("Wii-hab") provides benefits in Parkinson's disease. Parkinsonism & related disorders, 19(11), 1039-1042.

Hewett, T.E., Myer, G.D., Ford, K.R., Heidt, R.S. Jr., Colosimo, A.J., McLean, S.G., van den Bogert, A.J., Paterno, M.V., Succop, P. (2005). Biomechanical measures of neuromuscular control and valgus loading of the knee predict anterior cruciate ligament injury risk in female athletes: a prospective study. *The American journal of sports medicine. 33*(4):492-501.

Hilberg T., Hersbsleb M., Puta C., Gabriel H. H. W., Schramm W. (2003). Physical training increases isometric muscular strength and proprioceptive performance in haemophilic subjects. Haemophilia 9, 86–93. 10.1046/j.1365-2516.2003.00679.x

Hill, K. D., LoGiudice, D., Lautenschlager, N. T., Said, C. M., Dodd, K. J., & Suttanon, P. (2009). Effectiveness of balance training exercise in people with mild to moderate severity Alzheimer's disease: Protocol for a randomised trial. *BMC geriatrics*, 16(9), 29. Doi: 10.1186/1471-2318-9-29

Hill, K. D., Williams, S. B., Chen, J., Moran, H., Hunt, S., & Brand, C. (2013). Balance and falls risk in women with lower limb osteoarthritis or rheumatoid arthritis. Journal of Clinical Gerontology and Geriatrics, 4(1), 22-28.

Hirsch, M. A., Toole, T., Maitland, C. G., & Rider, R. A. (2003). The effects of balance training and high- intensity resistance training on persons with idiopathic Parkinson's disease. *Archives of physical medicine and rehabilitation*, *84*(8). 1109–17. Retrieved from http://www.marianjoylibrary.org/Residency/Focus/documents/Ref52.pdf

Hlavackova, P., Fristios, J., Cuisinier, R., Pinsault, N., Janura, M., & Vuillerme, N. (2009). Effects of mirror feedback on upright stance control in elderly transfemoral amputees. Archives of physical medicine and rehabilitation, 90(11), 1960-1963.

Hocherman S. (1993). Proprioceptive guidance and motor planning of reaching movements to unseen targets. Exp. Brain Res. 95, 349–358. 10.1007/BF00229793

Hocherman S., Aharonson D., Medalion B., Hocherman I. (1988). Perception of the immediate extrapersonal space through proprioceptive inputs. Exp. Brain Res. 73, 256–262. 10.1007/BF00248218

Hornbrook, M.C., Stevens, V.J., Wingfield, D.J., Hollis, J.F., Greenlick, M.R., Ory, M.G. (1994). Preventing falls among community-dwelling older persons: results from a randomized trial. *The Gerontologist. 34*(1):16-23.

Huisinga JM, Filipi ML, Stergiou N. Supervised resistance training results in changes in postural control in patients with multiple sclerosis. Motor control. Jan 2012;16(1):50-63.

Ilg, W., Giese, M. A., Gizewski, E. R., Schoch, B., & Timmann, D. (2008). The influence of focal cerebellar lesions on the control and adaptation of gait. *Brain : a journal of neurology, 131*(Pt 11), 2913–27. Doi: 10.1093/brain/awn246

Jackson K, Edginton-Bigelow K, Cooper C, Merriman H. A group kickboxing program for balance, mobility, and quality of life in individuals with multiple sclerosis: a pilot study. Journal of neurologic physical therapy : JNPT. Sep 2012;36(3):131-137.

Jacobson B. H., Chen H. C., Cashel C., Guerrero L. (1997). The effect of T'ai Chi Chuan training on balance, kinesthetic sense, and strength. Percept. Mot. Skills 84, 27–33. 10.2466/pms.1997.84.1.27

Jan M. H., Tang P. F., Lin J. J., Tseng S. C., Lin Y. F., Lin D. H. (2008). Efficacy of a target-matching foot-stepping exercise on proprioception and function in patients with knee osteoarthritis. J. Orthop. Sports Phys. Ther. 38, 19–25. 10.2519/jospt.2008.2512

Jogi, P., Overend, T. J., Spaulding, S. J., Zecevic, A., & Kramer, J. F. (2015). Effectiveness of balance exercises in the acute post-operative phase following total hip and knee arthroplasty: A randomized clinical trial. SAGE Open Medicine, 3, 2050312115570769.

Ju Y. Y., Wang C. W., Cheng H. Y. (2010). Effects of active fatiguing movement versus passive repetitive movement on knee proprioception. Clin. Biomech. 25, 708–712. 10.1016/j.clinbiomech.2010.04.017

Kaelin-Lang A., Sawaki L., Cohen L. G. (2005). Role of voluntary drive in encoding an elementary motor memory. J. Neurophysiol. 93, 1099–1103. 10.1152/jn.00143.2004

Kim, S. H., Wise, B. L., Zhang, Y., & Szabo, R. M. (2011). Increasing incidence of shoulder arthroplasty in the United States. The Journal of Bone & Joint Surgery, 93(24), 2249-2254.

Klages K., Zecevic A., Orange J. B., Hobson S. (2011). Potential of Snoezelen room multisensory stimulation to improve balance in individuals with dementia: a feasibility randomized controlled trial. Clin. Rehabil. 25, 607–616. 10.1177/0269215510394221

Konczak J., Corcos D. M., Horak F., Poizner H., Shapiro M., Tuite P., et al. . (2009). Proprioception and motor control in Parkinson's disease. J. Mot. Behav. 41, 543–552. 10.3200/35-09-002

Kurz, A., Pohl, C., Ramsenthaler, M., & Sorg, C. (2009). Cognitive rehabilitation in patients with mild cognitive impairment. *International journal of geriatric psychiatry, 24*(2), 163–8. Doi: 10.1002/gps.2086

Kurtz, S. M., Lau, E., Ong, K., Zhao, K., Kelly, M., & Bozic, K. J. (2009). Future young patient demand for primary and revision joint replacement: national projections from 2010 to 2030. Clinical Orthopaedics and Related Research, 467(10), 2606–12. doi:10.1007/s11999-009-0834-6

Kynsburg A., Halasi T., Tallay A., Berkes I. (2006). Changes in joint position sense after conservatively treated chronic lateral ankle instability. Knee Surg. Sports Traumatol. Arthrosc. 14, 1299–1306. 10.1007/s00167-006-0106-x

Kynsburg A., Panics G., Halasi T. (2010). Long-term neuromuscular training and ankle joint position sense. Acta Physiol. Hung. 97, 183–191. 10.1556/APhysiol.97.2010.2.4

Liao, C. D., Liou, T. H., Huang, Y. Y., & Huang, Y. C. (2013). Effects of balance training on functional outcome after total knee replacement in patients with knee osteoarthritis: a randomized controlled trial. Clinical rehabilitation, 27(8), 697-709.

Lin D. H., Lin C. H., Lin Y. F., Jan M. H. (2009). Efficacy of 2 non-weight-bearing interventions, proprioception training versus strength training, for patients with knee osteoarthritis: a randomized clinical trial. J. Orthop. Sports Phys. Ther. 39, 450–457. 10.2519/jospt.2009.2923

Lin D. H., Lin Y. F., Chai H. M., Han Y. C., Jan M. (2007). Comparison of proprioceptive functions between computerized proprioception facilitation exercise and closed kinetic chain exercise in patients with knee osteoarthritis. Clin. Rheumatol. 26, 520–528. 10.1007/s10067 006-0324-0

Liu S. Y., Hsieh C. L., Wei T. S., Liu P. T., Chang Y. J., Li T. C. (2009). Acupuncture stimulation improves balance function in stroke patients: a single-blinded controlled, randomized study. Am. J Chin. Med. 37, 483–494. 10.1142/S0192415X09006990

Lloyd, D. G. (2001). Rationale for training programs to reduce anterior cruciate ligament injuries in Australian football. Journal of Orthopaedic & Sports Physical Therapy, *31*(11), 645–654.

Lloyd, B. D., Williamson, D. A., Singh, N. A., Hansen, R. D., Diamond, T. H., Finnegan, T. P., ... & Singh, M. A. F. (2009). Recurrent and injurious falls in the year following hip fracture: a prospective study of incidence and risk factors from the Sarcopenia and Hip Fracture study. *The Journals of Gerontology Series A: Biological Sciences and Medical Sciences*, *64*(5), 599-609. http://biomedgerontology.oxfordjournals.org/content/64A/5/599.short

Lobstein, T. (2015). Prevalence and costs of obesity. Medicine, 43(2), 77–79. doi:10.1016/j.mpmed.2014.11.011

Lynch E. A., Hillier S. L., Stiller K., Campanella R. R., Fisher P. H. (2007). Sensory retraining of the lower limb after acute stroke: a randomized controlled pilot trial. Arch. Phys. Med. Rehabil. 88, 1101–1107. 10.1016/j.apmr.2007.06.010

Ma, H. I., Hwang, W. J., Wang, C. Y., Fang, J. J., Leong, I. F., & Wang, T. Y. (2012). Trunk–arm coordination in reaching for moving targets in people with Parkinson's disease: Comparison between virtual and physical reality. *Human movement science*, *31*(5), 1340-1352.

Mace M. J., Levin O., Alaerts K., Rothwell J. C., Swinnen S. P. (2008). Corticospinal facilitation following prolonged proprioceptive stimulation by means of passive wrist movement. J. Clin. Neurophysiol. 25, 202–209. 10.1097/WNP.0b013e31817da170

Mandelbaum, B. R., Silvers, H. J., Watanabe, D. S., Knarr, J. F., Thomas, S. D., Griffin, L.Y., Kirkendall, D.T., Garrett, W. Jr. (2005). Effectiveness of a neuromuscular and proprioceptive training program in preventing anterior cruciate ligament injuries in female athletes: 2-year follow-up. *The American journal of sports medicine*, *33*(7), 1003–10. Doi: 10.1177/0363546504272261

McGuine, T. A., Greene, J. J., Best, T., & Leverson, G. (2000). Balance as a predictor of ankle injuries in high school basketball players. *Clinical journal of sport medicine : official journal of the Canadian Academy of Sport Medicine*, *10*(4), 239–44.

McGuine, T. A., & Keene, J. S. (2006). The effect of a balance training program on the risk of ankle sprains in high school athletes. *The American journal of sports medicine*, *34*(7), 1103–11. Doi: 10.1177/0363546505284191

McHugh, M. P., Tyler, T. F., Mirabella, M. R., Mullaney, M. J., & Nicholas, S. J. (2007). The effectiveness of a balance training intervention in reducing the incidence of noncontact ankle sprains in high school football players. *The American journal of sports medicine*, *35*(8), 1289–1294. doi: 10.1177/0363546507300059

McKenzie A., Goldman S., Barrango C., Shrime M., Wong T., Byl N. (2009). Differences in physical characteristics and response to rehabilitation for patients with hand dystonia: musicians' cramp compared to writers' cramp. J. Hand Ther. 22, 172. 10.1016/j.jht.2008.12.006

Merkert J., Butz S., Nieczaj R., Steinhagen-Thiessen E., Eckardt R. (2011). Combined whole body vibration and balance training using vibrosphere: improvement of trunk stability, muscle tone, and postural control in stroke patients during early geriatric rehabilitation. Z. Gerontol. Geriatr. 44, 256–261. 10.1007/s00391-011-0170-9

Missaoui B., Thoumie P. (2009). How far do patients with sensory ataxia benefit from so-called "proprioceptive rehabilitation"? Neurophysiol. Clin. 39, 229–233. 10.1016/j.neucli.2009.07.002

Mohammadi, F. (2007). Comparison of 3 preventive methods to reduce the recurrence of ankle inversion sprains in male soccer players The American journal of sports medicine, *35*(6), 922–926. Doi: 10.1177/0363546507299259

Mutha, P. K., Boulinguez, P., & Sainburg, R. L. (2008). Visual modulation of proprioceptive reflexes during movement. *Brain Research*, *1246*(2008), 54–69. doi: 10.1016/j.brainres.2008.09.061

Myer, G. D., Brunner, H. I., Melson, P. G., Paterno, M. V., Ford, K. R., & Hewett, T. E. (2005). Specialized neuromuscular training to improve neuromuscular function and biomechanics in a patient with quiescent juvenile rheumatoid arthritis. *Physical therapy*, *85*(8), 791–802. Retrieved from ptjournal.apta.org/content/85/8/791.full

Myer, G. D., Ford, K. R., Brent, J. L., & Hewett, T. E. (2006). The effects of plyometric vs. dynamic stabilization and balance training on power, balance, and landing force in female athletes. *Journal of strength and conditioning research / National Strength & Conditioning Association*, *20*(2), 345–353. Doi: 10.1519/R-17955.1

Myer, G. D., Paterno, M. V., Ford, K. R., Quatman, C. E., & Hewett, T. E. (2006). Rehabilitation after anterior cruciate ligament reconstruction: Criteria-based progression through the return-to- sport phase. *The Journal of orthopaedic and sports physical therapy*, *36*(6), 385–402. Retrieved from www.jospt.org/members/getfile.asp?id=2455

Murillo, N., Valls-Sole, J., Vidal, J., Opisso, E., Medina, J., & Kumru, H. (2014). Focal vibration in neurorehabilitation. European journal of physical and rehabilitation medicine, 50(2), 231-242.

Olson, S. A., Furman, B., & Guilak, F. (2012). Joint injury and post-traumatic arthritis. HSS Journal : The Musculoskeletal Journal of Hospital for Special Surgery, 8(1), 23–5. doi:10.1007/s11420-011-9247-7

Paltamaa J, Sjogren T, Peurala SH, Heinonen A. Effects of physiotherapy interventions on balance in multiple sclerosis: a systematic review and meta-analysis of randomized controlled trials. Journal of rehabilitation medicine : official journal of the UEMS European Board of Physical and Rehabilitation Medicine. Oct 2012;44(10):811-823.

Panics, G., Tallay, A., Pavlik, A., & Berkes, I. (2008). Effect of proprioception training on knee joint position sense in female team handball players. *British journal of sports medicine*, *42*(6), 472–6. Doi: 10.1136/bjsm.2008.046516

Panics G., Tallay A., Pavlik A., Berkes I. (2008). Effect of proprioception training on knee joint position sense in female team handball players. Br. J. Sports Med. 42, 472–476. 10.1136/bjsm.2008.046516

Park, J. H., Cho, H., Shin, J. H., Kim, T., Park, S. B., Choi, B. Y., & Kim, M. J. (2014). Relationship among fear of falling, physical performance, and physical characteristics of the rural elderly. *American Journal of Physical Medicine & Rehabilitation*, *93*(5), 379-386.

Park JS, Lee D, Lee S *et al.* (2011). Comparison of the effects of aquatic and land exercise by chronic stroke patients. *J Phys Ther Sci, 23:* 821-824.

Patel, N., Hanfelt, J., Marsh, L., & Jankovic, J. (2014). Alleviating manoeuvres (sensory tricks) in cervical dystonia. Journal of Neurology, Neurosurgery & Psychiatry, jnnp-2013.

Paterno, M. V., Myer, G. D., Ford, K. R., & Hewett, T. E. (2004). Neuromuscular training improves single- limb stability in young female athletes. *The Journal of orthopaedic and sports physical therapy*, *34*(6), 305–316. Retrieved from www.jospt.org/members/getfile.asp?id=1943

Peterson EW, Ben Ari E, Asano M, Finlayson ML. Fall attributions among middle-aged and older adults with multiple sclerosis. Archives of physical medicine and rehabilitation. May 2013;94(5):890-895.

Picelli, A., Tamburin, S., Passuello, M., Waldner, A., & Smania, N. (2014). Robot-assisted arm training in patients with Parkinson's disease: a pilot study. *Journal of neuroengineering and rehabilitation*, *11*(28).

Porciuncula, F., Johnson, C. C., & Glickman, L. B. (2012). The effect of vestibular rehabilitation on adults with bilateral vestibular hypofunction: a systematic review. Journal of Vestibular Research, 22(5), 283.

Pozo-Cruz, B. D., Adsuar, J. C., Parraca, J. A., Pozo-Cruz, J. D., Olivares, P. R., & Gusi, N. (2012). Using whole-body vibration training in patients affected with common neurological diseases: a systematic literature review. *The Journal of Alternative and Complementary Medicine*, *18*(1), 29-41.

Prisk, G. (2012). The effectiveness of sensory integration to enhance occupational engagement in children with sensory process. Retrieved from http://www.nzaot.com/downloads/contribute/GPiskSIchildren.pdf

Protas, E. J., Mitchell, K., Williams, A., Qureshy, H., Caroline, K., & Lai, E. C. (2005). Gait and step training to reduce falls in Parkinson's disease. *NeuroRehabilitation*, *20*(3), 183–90. Retrieved from http://www.ncpad.org/545/2484/Gait~and~step~training~to~reduce~falls~in~Parkinson~s~disease

Ramos, V. F. M. L., Karp, B. I., & Hallett, M. (2014). Tricks in dystonia: ordering the complexity. Journal of Neurology, Neurosurgery & Psychiatry, 85(9), 987-993.

Ribeiro, T., Britto, H., Oliveira, D., Silva, E., Galvão, E., & Lindquist, A. (2013). Effects of treadmill training with partial body weight support and the proprioceptive neuromuscular facilitation method on hemiparetic gait: a randomized controlled study. *European journal of physical and rehabilitation medicine*, *49*(4), 451-461.

Robin C., Toussaint L., Blandin Y., Vinter A. (2004). Sensory integration in the learning of aiming toward "self- defined" targets. Res. Q. Exerc. Sport 75, 381–387. 10.1080/02701367.2004.10609171

Röijezon U., Björklund M., Bergenheim M., Djupsjöbacka M. (2009). A novel method for neck coordination exercise–a pilot study on persons with chronic non-specific neck pain. J. Neuroeng. Rehabil. 5:36. 10.1186/1743-0003-5-36

Rosenkranz K., Butler K., Williamon A., Cordivari C., Lees A. J., Rothwell J. C. (2008). Sensorimotor reorganization by proprioceptive training in musician's dystonia and writer's cramp. Neurology 70, 304–315. 10.1212/01.wnl.0000296829.66406.14

Rosenkranz K., Butler K., Williamon A., Rothwell J. C. (2009). Regaining motor control in musician's dystonia by restoring sensorimotor organization. J. Neurosci. 29, 14627–14636. 10.1523/JNEUROSCI.2094-09.2009

Rozzi, S. L., Lephart, S. M., Gear, W. S., & Fu, F. H. (1999). Knee joint laxity and neuromuscular characteristics of male and female soccer and basketball players. *The American journal of sports medicine*, *27*(3), 312–9. Retrieved from http://www.pitt. edu/~neurolab/publications/1999/Articles/RozziSL_1999_AmJSportsMed_Knee%20 joint%20laxity%20and%20neuromuscular%20characteristics%20of%20male%20and%20 female%20soccer%20and%20basketball%20players.pdf

Rubenstein, L. Z. (2006). Falls in older people: epidemiology, risk factors and strategies for prevention. *Age and ageing*, *35*(2), ii37-ii41.

Sahay, P., Prasad, S. K., Anwer, S., Lenka, P. K., & Kumar, R. (2014). Efficacy of proprioceptive neuromuscular facilitation techniques versus traditional prosthetic training for improving ambulatory function in transtibial amputees. Hong Kong Physiotherapy Journal, 32(1), 28-34.

Saposnik, G., & Levin, M. (2011). Virtual reality in stroke rehabilitation a meta-analysis and implications for clinicians. *Stroke*, *42*(5), 1380-1386.

Saverino, A., Benevolo, E., Ottonello, M., Zsirai, E., & Sessarego, P. (2006). Falls in a rehabilitation setting: functional independence and fall risk. *Europa medicophysica*, *42*(3), 179-184.

Schenkman, M., Hall, D., Kumar, R., & Kohrt, W. M. (2008). Endurance exercise training to improve economy of movement of people with Parkinson disease: Three case reports. *Physical Therapy*, *88*(1), 63–76. Retrieved from www.physther.org/content/88/1/63.full

Schiftan, G. S., Ross, L. A., & Hahne, A. J. (2015). The effectiveness of proprioceptive training in preventing ankle sprains in sporting populations: A systematic review and meta-analysis. *Journal of Science and Medicine in Sport*, *18*(3), 238-244.

Sekir U., Gür H. (2005). A multi-station proprioceptive exercise program in patients with bilateral knee osteoarthrosis: functional capacity, pain and sensoriomotor function. A randomized controlled trial. J. Sports Sci. Med. 4, 590–603.

Sherry, M. A., & Best, T. M. (2004). A comparison of 2 rehabilitation programs in the treatment of acute hamstring strains. *The Journal of orthopaedic and sports physical therapy*, *34*(3), 116–125. Retrieved from www.jospt.org/issues/articleID.260,type.2/article_detail. asp

Schmidt, J., Fleming, J., Ownsworth, T., & Lannin, N. A. (2012). Video Feedback on Functional Task Performance Improves Self-awareness After Traumatic Brain Injury A Randomized Controlled Trial. Smith, T. O., King, J. J., & Hing, C. B. (2012). The effectiveness of proprioceptive-based exercise for osteoarthritis of the knee: a systematic review and meta-analysis. Rheumatology international, 32(11), 3339-3351.

Schuster, C., Hilfiker, R., Amft, O., Scheidhauer, A., Andrews, B., Butler, J., ... & Ettlin, T. (2011). Best practice for motor imagery: a systematic literature review on motor imagery training elements in five different disciplines. BMC medicine, 9(1), 75.

Statista.com (2015). Projected worldwide increase in prevalence of Parkinson's disease in 2005 and 2030 (in million patients). Retrieved from http://www.statista.com/statistics/215459/projected-worldwide-increase-in-prevalence-of-parkinsons-diseas/

Statistic Brain Research Institute. (7/28/2013). Diabetes Amputation Prevention, Net Wellness. Retrieved from http://www.statisticbrain.com/amputee-statistics/

Statistic Brain Research Institute. (11/23/2013). Multiple sclerosis statistics. Retrieved from http://www.statisticbrain.com/multiple-sclerosis-statistics/

Statistic Brain Research Institute. (3/12/2015). Alzheimer's Association statistics. Retrieved from http://www.statisticbrain.com/alzheimers-disease-statistics/

Stevenson, T., Thalman, L., Christie, H., & Poluha, W. (2012). Constraint-induced movement therapy compared to dose-matched interventions for upper-limb dysfunction in adult survivors of stroke: a systematic review with meta-analysis. *Physiotherapy Canada*, *64*(4), 397-413.

Struppler A., Havel P., Müller-Barna P. (2003). Facilitation of skilled finger movements by repetitive peripheral magnetic stimulation (RPMS)-a new approach in central paresis. Neurorehabilitation 18, 69–82.

Sutoo, D., & Akiyama, K. (2003). Regulation of brain function by exercise. *Neurobiology of disease*, *13*(1), 1–14.

Sveistrup, H. (2004). Motor rehabilitation using virtual reality. Journal of NeuroEngineering and Rehabilitation, 1(10)

Swinnen, E., Beckwée, D., Meeusen, R., Baeyens, J. P., & Kerckhofs, E. (2014). Does robot-assisted gait rehabilitation improve balance in stroke patients? A systematic review. *Topics in stroke rehabilitation*, *21*(2), 87-100.

Swinnen, E., Beckwée, D., Pinte, D., Meeusen, R., Baeyens, J. P., & Kerckhofs, E. (2012). Treadmill training in multiple sclerosis: can body weight support or robot assistance provide added value? A systematic review. Multiple sclerosis international, 2012.

Telles, S., Hanumanthaiah, B., Nagarathna, R., & Nagendra, H. R. (1993). Improvement in static motor performance following yogic training of school children. *Perceptual and motor skills*, 76(3 Pt 2). 1264–6. Retrieved from http://katrinadurocher.com/files/kids_yoga_research_muscle.pdf

Teri, L., Gibbons, L. E., McCurry, S. M., Logsdon, R. G., Buchner, D.M., Barlow, W.E., Kukull, W.A., LaCroix, A.Z., McCormick, W., Larson, E.B. (2003). Exercise plus behavioral management in patients with Alzheimer disease: A randomized controlled trial. *JAMA : the journal of the American Medical Association*, 290(15). 2015–22. Doi: 10.1001/jama.290.15.2015

Teri, L., McCurry, S. M., Buchner, D. M., Logsdon, R. G., LaCroix, A. Z., Kukull, W.A., Barlow, W.E., Larson, E.B. (1998). Exercise and activity level in Alzheimer's disease: A potential treatment focus. *Journal of rehabilitation research and development*, 35(4), 411–9. Retrieved from http://www.rehabilitation.research.va.gov/jour/98/35/4/teri.pdf

Tsang, W. W., & Hui-Chan, C. W. (2004). Effect of 4- and 8-wk intensive Tai Chi Training on balance control in the elderly. *Medicine and science in sports and exercise*, 36(4), 648–57.

Thomas, R.H., Daniels, T.R (2003). Ankle arthritis. J Bone Joint Surg Am, 85-A(5):923-36

Van Delden, A. L. E. Q., Peper, C. L. E., Kwakkel, G., & Beek, P. J. (2012). A systematic review of bilateral upper limb training devices for poststroke rehabilitation. *Stroke research and treatment*, 2012.

van Nes I. J., Latour H., Schils F., Meijer R., van Kuijk A., Geurts A. C. (2006). Long-term effects of 6-week whole-body vibration on balance recovery and activities of daily living in the postacute phase of stroke: a randomized, controlled trial. Stroke 37, 2331–2335. 10.1161/01.STR.0000236494.62957.f3

van Nes I. J. W., Geurts A. C. H., Hendricks H. T., Duysens J. (2004). Short-term effects of whole-body vibration on postural control in unilateral chronic stroke patients. Am. J. Phys. Med. Rehabil. 83, 867–873. 10.1097/01.PHM.0000140801.23135.09

Vaugoyeau, M., Viel, S., Amblard, B., Azulay, J. P., & Assaiante, C. (2008). Proprioceptive contribution of postural control as assessed from very slow oscillations of the support in healthy humans. *Gait Posture*, 27(2), 294–302. Retrieved from http://www.gaitposture.com/article/S0966-6362(07)00108-7/fulltext

Vu, M. Q., Weintraub, N., & Rubenstein, L. Z. (2006). Falls in the nursing home: are they preventable? *Journal of the American Medical Directors Association, 7*(3), S53-S58. http://www.jamda.com/article/S1525-8610(05)00690-0/abstract

Weiss, P. L., Rand, D., Katz, N., & Kizony, R. (2004). Video capture virtual reality as a flexible and effective rehabilitation tool. Journal of neuroengineering and rehabilitation, 1(1), 12.

Wester, J. U., Jespersen, S. M., Nielsen, K. D., & Neumann, L. (1996). Wobble board training after partial sprains of the lateral ligaments of the ankle: A prospective randomized study. *The Journal of orthopaedic and sports physical therapy, 23*(5), 332–336. Retrieved from www.jospt.org/issues/articleID.977/article_detail.asp

Westlake K. P., Culham E. G. (2007). Sensory-specific balance training in older adults: effect on proprioceptive reintegration and cognitive demands. Phys. Ther. 87, 1274–1283. 10.2522/ptj.20060263

Wong J. D., Kistemaker D. A., Chin A., Gribble P. L. (2012). Can proprioceptive training improve motor learning? J. Neurophysiol. 108, 3313–3321. 10.1152/jn.00122.2012

Wong J. D., Wilson E. T., Gribble P. L. (2011). Spatially selective enhancement of proprioceptive acuity following motor learning. J. Neurophysiol. 105, 2512–2521. 10.1152/jn.00949.2010

Wright, N. C., Looker, A. C., Saag, K. G., Curtis, J. R., Delzell, E. S., Randall, S., & Dawson☒Hughes, B. (2014). The recent prevalence of osteoporosis and low bone mass in the United States based on bone mineral density at the femoral neck or lumbar spine. Journal of Bone and Mineral Research, 29(11), 2520-2526.

Yang, Y., Verkuilen, J. V., Rosengren, K. S., Grubisich, S. A., Reed, M. R., & Hsiao-Wecksler, E. T. (2007). Effect of combined Taiji and Qigong training on balance mechanisms: a randomized controlled trial of older adults. *Medical science monitor: international medical journal of experimental and clinical research, 13*(8), CR339–48.

Yilmaz I., Birkan B., et al. (2010). Effects of Constant Time Delay Procedure on the Halliwick's Method of Swimming Rotation Skills for Children with Autism. Education and Training in Autism and Developmental Disabilities, 45(1).

Yilmaz I., Birkan B., Konukman F., Erkan M. (2005). Using a Constant Time Delay Procedure to Teach Aquatic Play Skills to Children with Autism. Education and Training in Developmental Disabilities, 40(2).

You, S. H., Jang, S. H., Kim, Y. H., Kwon, Y. H., Barrow, I., & Hallett, M. (2005). Cortical reorganization induced by virtual reality therapy in a child with hemiparetic cerebral palsy. Developmental Medicine & Child Neurology, 47(09), 628-635.

Yozbatiran N., Donmez B., Kayak N., Bozan O. (2006). Electrical stimulation of wrist and fingers for sensory and functional recovery in acute hemiplegia. Clin. Rehabil. 20, 4–11. 10.1191/0269215506cr928oa

APPENDIX

Examination

Upon meeting the Satisfactory Completion Statement, you may receive a certificate of completion at the end of this course.

Contact ceu@rehabsurge.com to find out if this distance learning course is an approved course from your board. Save your course outline and contact your own board or organization for specific filing requirements.

In order to obtain continuing education hours, you must have read the book, have completed the exam and survey. Please include a $50.00 exam fee for your exam. Mail the exam answer sheet and survey sheet to:

Rehabsurge, Inc.
PO Box 287
Baldwin, NY 11510
Allow 2–4 weeks to receive your certificate.

You can also take the exam online at www.rehabsurge.com. Register and pay the exam fee of $50.00. After you passed the exam with a score of 70%, you will be able to print your certificate immediately. See rehabsurge.com for more details.

Exam Questions:

1. Balance control in humans is reliant upon:

    a. Visual cues

    b. Vestibular cues

    c. Cues coming from the entire muscular system

    d. Cues coming from the entire immune system

2. Which input is very important in maintaining balance and posture?

    a. Visual input

    b. Auditory input

    c. Tactile input

    d. Kinesiologic input

3. When do infants acquire adequate neck muscle control, enough to stabilize their head?

    a. 2 months

    b. 3 months

    c. 4 months

    d. 6 months

4. In this stage, when children begin to walk, what is deemed to be the important step?

    a. Stabilization of the neck

    b. Stabilization of the thoracic spine

    c. Stabilization of the pelvis

    d. Stabilization of the knees

5. In the case study by Mandelbaum et al 2005 with soccer players for proprioceptive training, over a two year period, the occurrence of anterior cruciate ligament injury was reduced by how many percentage points in the proprioceptive training group as compared to the control group?

    a. 75%

    b. 78%

    c. 85%

    d. 88%

6. Proprioceptive training strategies result in all of the following except:

   a. Enhanced balance

   b. Enhanced joint perception

   c. Increased ankle injuries and sprains

   d. Improved posture maintenance.

7. Dr. Heath and colleagues at the Utah State University, Logan, UT and Lamar University, Beaumont, Texas subjected the participants to tests for static balance. Static balance test included all of the following except:

   a. Double leg stance

   b. Single leg stance

   c. Tandem stance

   d. Heel raise stance

8. Which disease can cause chronic and repetitive inflammation of joints in children?

   a. Juvenile rheumatoid arthritis

   b. Scleroderma

   c. Scoliosis

   d. Duchenne muscular dystrophy

9. In a case reported by Timothy E Hewett and colleagues in *Physical Therapy* in 2005, a 10-year-old with a case history of JRA was treated with a specialized neuromuscular training protocol. The warm up included:

   a. Walking with intervals of running on the treadmill

   b. Maintaining single leg stance for 5 minutes

   c. Heel to toe walking for 20 feet

   d. Negotiating 4 inch steps

10. In the same study above, they employed different components to their proprioceptive training protocol. Which of the following components are not used?

   a. Core Strengthening

   b. Endurance Training

   c. Unanticipated Training

   d. Landing Stance Correction

11. Participants who underwent yoga training demonstrated an increase in the maximum voluntary contraction force with the knee extensors by how many percentage points?

    a. 11%

    b. 12%

    c. 13%

    d. 14%

12. Exercise is known to increase the levels of:

    a. Endorphins

    b. Norepinephrine

    c. Bradykinin

    d. Substance P

13. Dr. Buchman and colleagues examined the correlations between daily physical activity and cognitive functions of elderly people not suffering from dementia. Which type of exercise proved to be most beneficial?

    a. Core strengthening

    b. Low impact exercise

    c. Heavy lifting

    d. Endurance training

14. Patients with mild cognitive impairment (MCI) were treated with combined approach of group activity planning, assertiveness training, stress management memory training and motor exercise. Following four weeks of therapy, patients with MCI showed significant improvements in performing:

    a. Daily living tasks

    b. Gait

    c. Distance running

    d. Lifting heavy objects

15. Parkinson's Disease patients with moderately advanced stage of disease were recruited in a gait training program. Patients were stabilized with safety harnesses onto treadmills and were asked to walk in all four directions (sideways, forwards and backwards). The training was carried out for

a. An hour, thrice a week for 2 weeks

b. An hour, thrice a week for 4 weeks

c. An hour, thrice a week for 6 weeks

d. An hour, thrice a week for 8 weeks

16. This exercise required a person to stand on one leg, say the left leg. The right leg is then raised such that the thigh is parallel to the ground and the knee is bent. The leg is then stretched forward such that the leg is now fully extended and parallel to the ground. Flexing the right hip, the leg is to be extended backward until the heel can point towards the buttocks. The right knee should then be flexed to bring the leg back to the ground.

a. Single leg stance

b. Bicycle swings

c. Toe walking

d. Heel walking

17. According to the model proposed by Dr. Christine Assaiante, stabilization of the head and neck is task dependent but pelvic stabilization is an integral part of all activities that children can perform up to the age of 6-7 years. Which exercise will be best?

a. Jumping through tires

b. Playing catch

c. Running

d. Negotiating stairs

18. This type of training requires sudden changes forcing reactionary loads on the patient's leg joints (within safe limits). This training protocol akin to maneuvers that the athlete would encounter in sport-specific training. These include sprinting and cutting drills.

a. Limb symmetry

b. Warm up

c. Unanticipated training

d. Core strengthening

19. Yoga sessions conducted for 75 minutes every day were found to improve proprioception. These sessions included all of the following except:

    a. Loosening (stretching) exercises for 5 minutes

    b. Breathing exercises for 10 minutes

    c. Physical postures (aka asanas) for 20 minutes

    d. Involuntary unregulated breathing (pranayama) for 10 minutes

20. Although women show a greater capability to balance on one leg, they display a time lag in sensing knee joint movement. This lack of proprioception seems to be compensated by greater activation of which muscle (as compared to men) when completing tasks like landing after a jump?

    a. Quadriceps

    b. Hamstrings

    c. Gluteus maximus

    d. Gastrocsoleus

ANSWER SHEET

Name:_____

Address:_____

Profession:_____

License Number:_____

Date:_____

E-mail Address (optional):_____

1. a b c d   11. a b c d

2. a b c d   12. a b c d

3. a b c d   13. a b c d

4. a b c d   14. a b c d

5. a b c d   15. a b c d

6. a b c d   16. a b c d

7. a b c d   17. a b c d

8. a b c d   18. a b c d

9. a b c d   19. a b c d

10. a b c d   20. a b c d

Please mail $50.00 and completed form to:

CEU Certificate Request

Rehabsurge, Inc.
PO Box 287
Baldwin, NY 11510.
Contact Us at:
Phone: +1 (516) 515-1267
Email: ceu@rehabsurge.com

Alternatively, you can take the exam online at www.rehabsurge.com

You will receive your certificate instantly.

It is the learner's responsibility to comply with all state and national regulatory board's rules and regulations. This includes but is not limited to:

- verifying and complying with applicable continuing education requirements;

- verifying and complying with all applicable standards of practice;

- verifying and complying with all licensure requirements;

- any other rules or laws identified in the learners state or regulatory board that is not mentioned here.

It is the learner's responsibility to complete ALL coursework in order to receive credit. This includes but is not limited to:

- Reading all course materials fully;

- Completing all course activities to meet the criteria set forth by the instructor;

- Completing and passing all applicable tests and quizzes. All learner's MUST take a comprehensive online exam where they MUST get at least 70%. Getting 70% is a requirement to pass.

IMPORTANT: Rehabsurge reserves the right to deny continuing education credits or withdraw credits issued at any time if: Coursework is found to be incomplete; It is determined that a user falsified, copied, and/or engaged in any flagrant attempt to manipulate, modify, or alter the coursework just to receive credit; and/or It is determined that the coursework was not completed by the user.

If any of the conditions above are determined, Rehabsurge reserves the right to notify any applicable state and national boards along with supporting documentation.

PROGRAM EVALUATION FORM

Rehabsurge, Inc. works to develop new programs based on your comments and suggestions, making your feedback on the program very important to us. We would appreciate you taking a few moments to evaluate this program.

Course Start Date:_____ Course End Date: _____

Course Start Time:_____ Course End Time:_____

Identity Verification: Name:_____

Profession:_____ License Number:_____State: _____

Please initial to indicate that you are the individual who read the book and completed the test. Initial here:_____

May we use your comments and suggestions in
upcoming marketing materials?   Yes   No

Would you take another seminar from Rehabsurge, Inc.?   Yes   No

The educational level required to read the book is: Beginner   Intermediate   Advanced

The course is:	(5-Yes/Excellent)			(1-No/Poor)	
Relevant to my profession	5	4	3	2	1
Valuable to my profession	5	4	3	2	1
Content matched stated objectives	5	4	3	2	1
Complete coverage of materials	5	4	3	2	1

Teaching ability	5	4	3	2	1
Organization of material	5	4	3	2	1
Effective	5	4	3	2	1

Please rate the objectives. After reading the material, how well do you feel you are able to meet?

Objective 1	5	4	3	2	1
Objective 2	5	4	3	2	1
Objective 3	5	4	3	2	1
Objective 4	5	4	3	2	1
Objective 5	5	4	3	2	1

What was the most beneficial part of the program? What was the least beneficial part of the program? _____

_____

_____

What would you like to see added to the program? In what ways might we make this program experience better for you?_____

_____

_____

If you have any general comments on this topic or program please explain. _____

_____

_____

_____

Please tell us what other programs or topics might interest you? _____

_____

_____

_____

Thank you for participating and taking the time to join us today!

50618740R00070

Made in the USA
Lexington, KY
23 March 2016